EXCESS CaLCIUM DISEASE

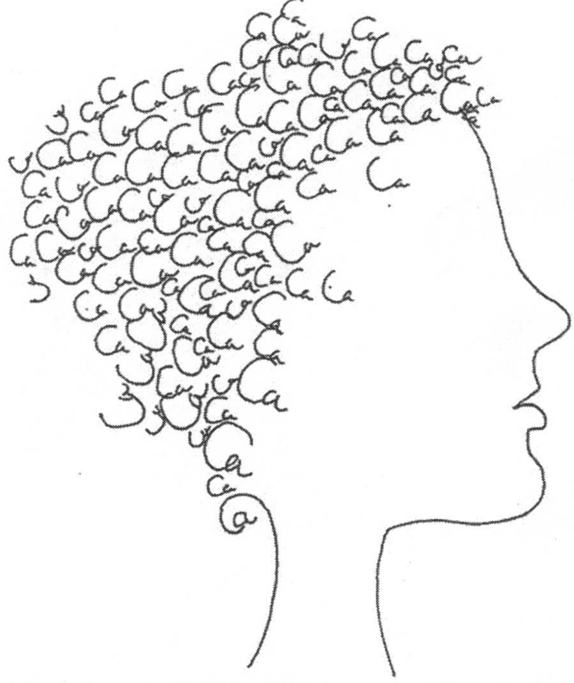

What you should know about high blood calcium, parathyroid hormone and hyperparathyroidism

Peter A. Galbraith

Published by Peter A. Galbraith 2015

excesscalciumdisease@gmail.com

Book formatting by BookCoverCafe.com

First Edition 2015

ISBN:
978-0-9906076-2-5 (pbk)
978-0-9906076-3-2 (ebk)

Cover illustration by Catherine Chapman Hess

Contents

Preface v

Nothing Should Be Done—? 1

Definitions for this Book 14

Do I (or Does Someone Close to Me) Have Excess Calcium Disease? 18

Symptoms—Should I Get a Blood Test? 33

Monitoring or Surgery? 53

Should I See an Endocrinologist? 66

Surgery and Selecting a Surgeon 79

Post-surgery Experience 99

About the Author 117

Preface

Hyperparathyroidism or excess calcium disease is one of the most under-diagnosed medical conditions in America with an estimated 3 million sufferers, 75% of whom are women. Experts estimate that half of America's primary care physicians do not properly diagnose the disease. Three of four women sufferers do not know they have it.

High calcium disease is often mistaken for simple aging. It is not! Common symptoms include chronic fatigue (frequent naps), excessive irritability, low mood (even depression), feeling miserable, and generally missing "the joy of life."

Excess calcium disease is an objective condition. You have it if you are over age 35 and your blood test shows calcium higher than 10.0. (75% of labs list too high a range for acceptable calcium levels!) In 80% of cases, you will also have a high parathyroid hormone level (PTH). No blood test? You can get a calcium blood test at a walk-in lab for under $30 without a doctor.

The high blood calcium is caused by a non-cancerous tumor growing on one (or more) of your four parathyroid glands. This tumor causes the secretion of too much parathyroid hormone, which, in turn, leaches calcium from your bones, weakening them. The excess calcium in your blood is deposited throughout your body. Left untreated, you can expect to suffer from chronic fatigue, low mood or depression, serious physical ailments like kidney stones and brittle bones, and a shortened life expectancy. The longer you have the disease, the more damage it does to your body and your mind.

Excess calcium disease is 100% cured by removal of the gland and tumor through outpatient surgery, the cost of which is covered by Medicare and all forms of private health insurance. There is no need to consult a specialist like an endocrinologist—you can self-refer to a parathyroid surgeon. Expect to feel 20 years younger after surgery!

Nothing Should Be Done—?

In mid-October, 2013, I was due to visit my primary care physician (PCP) for an annual physical examination. I had been seeing this doctor for fifteen years. We were both in our mid-60s and former runners and I liked his no-nonsense, blunt manner. Because an annual physical was expressly **not** covered by my private health insurance, these yearly visits were usually referenced as checkups for blood pressure medication. No matter the label, the routine was the same. After fasting overnight, I was to get a blood test in advance of my medical appointment and to show up for the examination after the results were in hand.

October 3, 2013 journal entry: "[At my upcoming physical], I'm going to get reamed as I am fat and out of shape, the worst I have ever been. Wasn't much I could do about it this summer or, if there was, I didn't do it."

Oct. 7. First blood test.

This year was different. After receiving the results of the blood test, my doctor requested a second blood test before my appointment. Although I live on an island with no ferry stop and it is a long and expensive trip to the mainland, I got the second test as requested.

Oct. 10. Second blood test.

During the October 15 physical, I was candid with my doctor. The summer had been "bad." My complaints were not earth shattering—frequent (even daily) naps in mid-afternoon, excess thirst and urination, general malaise. I was not hesitant to describe my months in Washington's San Juan Islands, which approach paradise during summer, as "bad." I wanted to communicate my low mood. I did not know what, if anything, was wrong, but I did not want to pretend things were okay.

At the exam, the mystery of the second blood test was soon explained. My first blood test showed a high level of calcium. The year before I had a high reading of calcium, too, but this year's level was really high. In this circumstance, the protocol called for my doctor to order a second blood test to measure the level of parathyroid hormone (PTH) in my blood. This result was also very high.

Okay, so I had high blood calcium. Interesting, I guess, but what did this mean and what was to be done? "Nothing," said my doctor.

He explained that during medical school he had learned about the "stones, bones, groans, and moans" syndrome. High calcium, he had been taught, was not a serious problem. It was not cancerous and while it could produce symptoms (of kidney stones, brittle bones, stomach groans, and psychic moans), the surgery to cure it presented such high risks that it was best not to do anything.

What were these risks? Primarily injury to the vocal cords (loss of voice) and possible removal of all four parathyroid glands or the entire thyroid, requiring one to take medication (not described) for the rest of one's life. Considering these risks, his advice was that nothing should be done.

I quizzed him further only about excess urination. I explained that during one 60-minute television show, I had to go to the bathroom, urgently, three times. This did not seem normal and could be distressing in social situations. "Drink less water," he told me.

My journal entry at the time recorded the physical this way: "Physical was fine. My weight was down from last year (!!) and my blood test results were down also, all of them, except for high calcium. Nothing can be done about high calcium that is worth doing . . . . As to being thirsty all the time and pissing too much, [my doctor] said, 'drink less water.'"

In fact, I left the physical feeling cheerful. My weight and my cholesterol levels were down from a year earlier. This high calcium thing was apparently nothing serious (it was not cancer). And despite being in the worst physical shape of my life, I had escaped without a chewing out, which my doctor was certainly entitled to give me.

On the same day as my physical, I drove with Cathy, who was travelling with me, to Sea-Tac airport, where we flew to Ft. Lauderdale, Florida. Two days later, we boarded a cruise ship, Holland America's Zaandam, for a month long voyage through the Panama Canal, down the Pacific coast of South America, around Cape Horn, and then north to Buenos Aires. While boarding the ship in Ft. Lauderdale, we met a couple, Dave and Carolyn, from the small town where I had my physical. Within a few days, we all ate dinner together in the Zaandam's dining room.

At that dinner, Carolyn said that she had recently had surgery for high blood calcium. She pointed to a thin, faint scar about 4" long running horizontally across her neck. (It looked to me just like a normal neck wrinkle.) When she mentioned high calcium, I brought up the results of my recent blood tests. Carolyn said that her surgery completely cured her condition (it is a disease) and resulted in an immediate and almost miraculous turnaround in her life. Her husband, Dave, agreed wholeheartedly.

Carolyn said that she had grown more and more irritable ("bitchy") and less and less energetic. When the two of them needed to pick up a few grocery items, for example, she would stay in the car and nap, while Dave did the actual shopping. She had surgery about four weeks before the wedding of her only daughter. According to Carolyn, when she awoke from surgery, her irritability was gone, her energy had fully returned, and she dove into wedding preparations with abandon. Moreover, the immediate improvement in energy level and elimination of symptoms proved to be permanent. She looked back on the time she suffered with high calcium disease with regret and wished she had not lost so much time from her life.

When the cruise was over, I immediately went on the Internet to learn what I could about high blood calcium. Google's number one search result was the parathyroid.com website sponsored by the Norman Parathyroid Center in Tampa, Florida. From that expansive website, I soon learned the basics of the disease. These were well presented and concisely explained in a five minute animated video, also available on YouTube.[1] Rather than summarize its contents, a complete transcript of the video follows:

Voiceover:

Hyperparathyroidism is a disease of the parathyroid glands affecting 1 in 800 people during their lifetime (graphic corrects this to 1 in 100 people) and 1 in 250 women over age 50 (graphic corrects this to 1 in 50 women over age 50).

Since parathyroid glands control the levels of calcium in our bodies, hyperparathyroidism is a disease of improper calcium regulation.

There are 4 parathyroid glands located behind the thyroid gland. Parathyroid glands monitor and control the amount of calcium in our blood and bones by secreting a hormone called parathyroid hormone or PTH. Each gland monitors the blood calcium and responds by making more or less PTH hormone.

1 As of this writing in early 2015, this video has 350,000 views on YouTube.

Hyperparathyroidism is a disease that occurs when one of the parathyroid glands develops a tumor. This tumor produces far too much parathyroid hormone, which is released into the bloodstream. The excess parathyroid hormone travels through the blood and into the bones. The hormone activates cells within the bones to eat away at the bones often causing osteoporosis, fractures and bone pain. The destruction of bone releases calcium into the blood. High blood calcium levels are seen in almost all patients with a parathyroid tumor.

The excess calcium can build up in the arteries, increasing atherosclerosis throughout the body. This can lead to high blood pressure and increased risks for heart attack and stroke. The high calcium often affects the electrical system of the heart, causing atrial fibrillation and palpitations.

The excess blood calcium builds up in the kidneys forming kidney stones and occasionally causing kidney failure.

High calcium levels also affect the brain. Since we use calcium in the electrical system of our nerves, a high blood calcium is associated with a slower nervous system, which gives symptoms of tiredness, memory loss, and poor concentration. Many patients with high blood calcium have chronic fatigue for this reason.

High calcium levels have an effect on the stomach and intestines often causing gastro esophageal reflux disease also known as GERD and abdominal discomfort.

High blood calcium is even associated with higher risks of several cancers including breast, prostate, colon, and kidney, some of which are more than twice as common in patients with high blood calcium.

It is estimated that untreated hyperparathyroidism can decrease a patient's life expectancy by 5 or 6 years even when the calcium is only slightly elevated.

There are no drugs, pills, or other treatments that can slow the process of bone destruction or take the place of surgical removal of the parathyroid tumor.

Hyperparathyroidism is cured by surgical removal of the parathyroid tumor. In the hands of an expert, parathyroid surgery is a straightforward outpatient procedure that can often be completed in less than 20 minutes. Since as many as 30% of patients with hyperparathyroidism will have more than one parathyroid tumor, your surgeon will examine all 4 parathyroid glands to be sure a second tumor has not been left behind.

Once all parathyroid tumors have been removed, the disease is cured. The process of eating away at the bones stops within minutes. The bone pain is typically gone within a few hours. The bones begin to regenerate within days and the osteoporosis begins to improve. The excess calcium in the blood will be gone within a few hours and within a week or two most patients feel significantly better. The health risks of high blood calcium begin diminishing within days of parathyroid tumor removal.

Hyperparathyroidism is a disease that typically makes people feel bad while it slowly destroys their body. All patients with hyperparathyroidism should be evaluated for a straightforward operation to remove the parathyroid tumor. Curing this disease has a tremendous impact on a patient's overall health and their quality of life.

End of voiceover.

Notwithstanding my increased knowledge about noncancerous tumors growing on rice-sized parathyroid glands, something about the parathyroid.com site bothered me. I remembered anecdotes about surgeons who always want to operate, to cut, as if that would solve everything. "Get Surgery" was a large part of the Norman Center's message. The parathyroid.com website even included a video of the surgery in question. It took less than 15 minutes, resulted in removal of two tumors from parathyroid glands (all four of which were checked and measured), achieved a complete cure, and left a scar only 1" in size (able to be hidden by a common band aid) that would disappear completely on healing.

It sounded too good to be true. Clearly, though, there were things going on that my own doctor had not mentioned. What to do?

Earlier I had called my doctor's office to ask for copies of my last three years of lab results. Now I decided to write a letter. My December 6 letter to my doctor began: "On my cruise, I met other folk who suffered from high calcium and had simple outpatient surgery on their parathyroid glands to remove a small tumor. This resulted in an immediate decrease (to normal) in the calcium level and a significant increase in energy." The letter continued: "Apparently the symptoms of which I complained in October ("bad summer," excess urination, and so forth) are consistent with hyperparathyroidism. Or perhaps I have medical student's disease."

I referenced the main claims on the Norman Center website, including that "parathyroid disease is the cause of high calcium at least 99.8% of the time" and that all that is needed for diagnosis is to measure blood calcium and parathyroid hormone (PTH) levels. I explained that I was considering outpatient surgery to remove the parathyroid tumor(s) and closed the letter by saying I was happy to discuss whether surgery "is appropriate or if this doctor is a quack."

My doctor called within a week. In our telephone conversation, he reviewed what he considered to be the risks of parathyroid surgery, including what he thought was a 5 to 7% chance of damage to the vocal cords and losing one's voice. When I observed that there were risks in not having the surgery, he agreed. His ultimate advice was that outpatient surgery was "not inappropriate."

My letter had mentioned a referral and my doctor offered to put me in touch with local surgeons, but I declined. I decided to self-refer to the Norman Center in Tampa. Information on the Center's website stated unequivocally that excess calcium disease (primary hyperparathyroidism) is an objective condition and that all health insurance companies and Medicare would pay for curative surgery, no questions asked. Self-referrals were encouraged and welcome.

There was only one hitch. The Norman Center appeared to contain the nation's leading parathyroid surgeons and experts in parathyroid disease. The website clarified that the surgeons would accept as full payment whatever amount Medicare (or a private insurer) would approve for the surgery. As I was recently eligible for Medicare, this was wonderful news. It appears that because of a willingness to accept minimal compensation for the surgery (at least from Medicare), the Norman Center doctors charged $1750 for a "one time" consultation before surgery could be scheduled. It was made clear that this "consultation fee" was not a proper charge against medical insurance or Medicare; it was labeled as a fee for which there could be no reimbursement from insurance or Medicare.

Three years of blood tests from my PCP arrived by snail mail. I spent $6 at Apple's App Store for the "Calcium Pro App" for my iPad. (It is also available online from calciumpro.com.) After entering my blood test results for three years, I clicked on the "Hyperparathyroid Analysis" button. On a scale from "very unlikely" on the left of the dial to "very likely" on the right, the needle pegged to the far right of the dial, to the extreme edge of the "very likely" category. Yep, I had excess calcium disease.

I contacted the Norman Center by email and paid the consultation fee by Visa over the telephone. I scanned my three years of blood test results into my computer and emailed them to the clinic. As the Norman Center closed for two weeks over Christmas, I felt lucky to complete a telephonic consultation with one of the surgeons before vacation began. The doctor reviewed my blood test results and declared it to be an open and shut case. He recommended surgery, adding, "If it was me, I would come to Tampa to get surgery." Yes, I said, that is what I intend to do.

I had surgery in Tampa from Dr. Norman and Dr. Politz on Tuesday, January 28, 2014. My life has improved markedly since then. Like Carolyn, I look back with regret on the time wasted while I endured excess calcium disease. During the Tampa surgery, I was told that I had suffered from excess calcium disease for 8 to 10 years. I will never get those years back.

I have not returned to my PCP since my surgery. The reason is simple. My doctor let me down. He gave me bad medical advice. Yet as I have further investigated excess calcium disease, I have learned that my doctor's response to the high calcium levels in my blood—do nothing!—is typical. It is likely that many, even most, primary care physicians in America would recommend the same as my doctor.

Dr. Norman has recently written that most family doctors in America are not capable of diagnosing primary hyperparathyroidism, or high calcium disease, and do not diagnose it. Even doctors who recognize excess calcium disease (did my doctor?) often recommend doing nothing about it. "Nothing should be done." This is wrong.

Many people suffer from excess calcium disease. If the parathyroid.com video is correct that 1% of the U.S. population suffers from it, then 3,200,000 people have primary hyperparathyroidism. Very few of them know it. **Three out of four patients with excess calcium disease are women. Dr. Norman has stated that three out of four women who have high calcium disease do not know it.** What a shame!

Immediately before my annual physical examination, my assessment of my condition was that I was "fat and out of shape, the worst I have ever been." The remainder of my October 3 journal entry apportions the blame—to me.

"[There] wasn't much I could do about it this summer or, if there was, I didn't do it." I expect that almost all people who suffer from high calcium disease blame themselves for how bad they feel and are frustrated and demoralized by their inability to do anything about it.

What is most troubling, however, is the realization that I could still be suffering from excess calcium disease. Had I not had dinner with Carolyn on the cruise ship, I do not think that I would have had surgery even today. Carolyn has told me that I am the only person she has ever met who had high blood calcium. Besides Carolyn, I have met only one other person with the disease. (Walter's story, told in a later chapter, is even more remarkable than Carolyn's or mine.)

This book is written partly as a public service to help readers learn the basics of excess calcium disease. The aim is to provide essential and current information about the disease and the treatment options available. I am not a doctor and the reader follows my "advice" at her peril. In this instance, however, it may be beneficial to read a disinterested layperson's analysis of the medical treatment currently available. This book is intended to help a person suffering from high calcium disease to recognize the disease, to make intelligent decisions regarding treatment, and, most important, to get appropriate medical care promptly, without wasting years of what could be a more active and happier life.

Action Items for Readers

1. Expect your doctor not to be familiar with excess calcium disease or modern surgical techniques to cure it.
2. Act as your own medical advisor regarding high calcium disease. Use this book and the Internet to make the correct decisions for your medical care.
3. From this book, learn what is a high blood calcium level and what is a normal blood calcium level. Be aware that many doctors apply too high a range for what is "normal" blood calcium.
4. Learn the symptoms of excess calcium disease. If you have any inkling that you have the disease, check the calcium level in your latest blood test. Or get an inexpensive current blood test (under $30) without involving your doctor.
5. If you have excess calcium disease, learn how to pick a surgeon and how to avoid delays in having the surgery needed to cure your disease.
6. Keep reading.

Definitions for this Book

Calcium glands are so important that nature provides them in quadruplicate—we only need one to function properly but we are given four to be certain that we have one that works. When a calcium gland is not functioning properly, when it has a non-cancerous tumor, too much calcium hormone is secreted resulting in too much calcium being leached from our bones with the result that the level of calcium in our blood is too high. When this happens, we have excess calcium disease or high calcium disease. It is cured by surgically removing the non-cancerous tumor(s) on the calcium gland(s).

These are simple concepts but the medical profession uses unnecessarily big words to explain them. This makes it difficult to understand what is going on and harder to make the correct choices. The names and descriptions used in connection with hyperparathyroidism (excess calcium disease) are a perfect example of needless obfuscation and the confusion that results. Dr. Norman wrote in a Norman Center blog on 11/13/13: "One of the things I would change if I could turn back time a few hundred years is the naming of parathyroid glands.

First, I wouldn't call them 'parathyroid glands.' I would give them a different name that wasn't confused with the thyroid."

Indeed, the problem starts with the parathyroid gland. This rice-sized (sometimes pea-sized) gland is so named because it is usually located near the thyroid gland. "Para" means beside or near. (Go ahead—check your dictionary.) The four glands that control the body's calcium levels are located near but have nothing to do with the function of the thyroid gland.[2] The name of these glands, parathyroid, causes much confusion. When I told my new doctor that I had recently had surgery to remove a parathyroid tumor, he ordered tests of my thyroid. When I asked him, gently, what he knew about hyperparathyroidism or excess calcium disease, he replied that he was required to refer a patient with high blood calcium to an endocrinologist. End of knowledge. Even now, one year after surgery, my new doctor orders tests to check the functioning of my thyroid gland in addition to testing calcium levels.

To better understand excess calcium disease, in this book relevant body parts are labeled by function, not by their medical name.

- Parathyroid gland is replaced by calcium gland. There are four.
- Parathyroid hormone (PTH) is replaced by calcium hormone (PTH).
- Primary hyperparathyroidism is replaced by either excess calcium disease or high calcium disease.

---

2 This book does not explain what the thyroid gland does because it is not relevant to anything about high calcium disease.

These are used interchangeably and mean exactly the same.

- Adenoma is a medical term referring to a non-cancerous tumor. As essentially all tumors growing on calcium glands are non-cancerous, adenoma is replaced by tumor.
- Parathyroidectomy normally refers to the surgery performed to remove adenomas or non-cancerous tumors growing on the calcium glands. It is replaced by calcium gland surgery.
- Carcinoma of the parathyroid gland, meaning cancer of the calcium gland, is so rare that it is not considered in this book.[3]
- Secondary hyperparathyroidism refers to a rare condition found usually in kidney dialysis patients. It should not concern the reader and will not be mentioned again. Tertiary hyperparathyroidism, a subset of secondary hyperparathyroidism, also will not be mentioned in this book. If you have either, stop reading this book.

To illustrate why these definitions are used, compare the following sentences. Using medical language, "primary hyperparathyroidism is always caused by adenoma(s) on the

3 Of more than 21,000 surgeries for excess calcium disease at the Norman Parathyroid Center, only 3 cases related to cancer of the calcium gland. Norman Center blog dated 6/21/13 written by Dr. Politz. If your doctor tells you that she wants to conduct tests to determine if you have a cancerous calcium gland, tell her no. The risk of cancer is nil but the tests your doctor may perform are unnecessary and can be dangerous.

parathyroid gland(s) and is cured by a parathyroidectomy performed by an endocrine surgeon (usually)." In this book's terminology, "excess calcium disease or high calcium disease is the result of a non-cancerous tumor on the calcium gland and is cured by calcium gland surgery performed by an expert in such surgery."

Please pay attention to this. Because medical professionals always use medical terminology, quotations in this book from medical doctors and medical websites are altered **without permission** to substitute this book's terminology. These changes are made so the lay reader can more easily understand the content of the quotation. Be assured that in early 2015, you will not hear or read of a medical person referring to a "calcium gland." In this book, you will not read further about a "parathyroid gland." The only exception is continued use of "PTH level." This refers to the calcium hormone level or parathyroid hormone level. "PTH level" is retained to assist the reader in interpreting lab test results, which list parathyroid hormone level or PTH level, not "calcium hormone level."

If you are a medical doctor, these definitions and use of this terminology may drive you crazy. These changes are made because the target audience for this book is a person with high blood calcium, not the doctor who treats her.

Lastly, the terms family doctor and primary care physician (or PCP) are used interchangeably to refer to the doctor first seen by a person with excess calcium disease. It is the family doctor or PCP who typically fails to diagnose high calcium disease.

Do I (or Does Someone Close to Me) Have Excess Calcium Disease?

Although excess calcium disease causes many subjective symptoms, making its sufferers miserable, the disease itself is an objective condition. In 99.8% of cases, high calcium disease is caused by a non-cancerous tumor growing on one or more of the four calcium glands. A tumor is either there or it is not. The presence of a calcium gland tumor is able to be reliably determined through objective lab tests. If one or more tumors are present, the level of calcium in the blood is too high. In addition, 80% of the time the level of calcium hormone (PTH) is also too high.

As high calcium disease is an objective condition, the question of whether one has the disease should be a simple inquiry, a yes or no question. The two key factors—a high blood calcium level and a high calcium hormone (PTH) level—are both able to be measured precisely. In 80% of cases of excess calcium disease, high levels of both are present.

In 20% of cases, sufferers have high blood calcium but not a high PTH level. Unfortunately, the absence of a high PTH level often leads PCPs to conclude that excess calcium disease is not present, especially if the blood calcium level is slightly higher than the normal range. Note that the simplicity of this analysis—an examination of two objective lab test measures—is the basis of the Calcium Pro App available for $6 on-line. Again, I entered my lab test results (and nothing else about symptoms), clicked on the "Hyperparathyroid Analysis" button, and watched the needle peg to the extreme right, confirming that I had excess calcium disease. It should be this simple for everyone and this chapter will help it be this simple for you.

What Is High Blood Calcium?

Given that a high calcium hormone (PTH) level is absent almost 20% of the time, the most reliable objective symptom of excess calcium disease is high blood calcium. What blood calcium level is normal and what is high?

Normal blood calcium levels vary depending upon age. In the teenage years, when our bodies are growing rapidly, especially our bones, normal levels of blood calcium can be as high as 10.7. In fact, for a 15 year old, a reading of 10.7 is not "high." For an adult, it is. **"Unfortunately very few doctors understand that the normal range for blood calcium changes as we age."** [emphasis in original] Norman Center blog (hereafter "NC blog") written by Dr. Norman, 7/11/13. (All NC blog entries are written by Dr. Norman unless otherwise noted.)

For middle-aged adults (over age 35), what is a high blood calcium level? The answer from Dr. Norman is a calcium level of 10.0 mg/dl or above. Put another way, the Norman Center advises that blood calcium readings for adults over age 35 "should be in the 9s." Adults over 40 "are not allowed to have calcium levels 'in the 10's' (rarely is ok, but not frequently, and not over 10.2)." Almost all adults over 35 should have calcium levels between 9.4 and 9.7 with 9.7 being the most common level. (same blog)

Many laboratories that report blood test results do not correlate the normal range for blood calcium to the patient's age. According to the Norman Center, as of mid-2013, at least 75% of blood test results list the wrong "normal range" for blood calcium. NC blog, 6/23/13. The upper limit of the normal range is always too high or above 10.0.

After reading this blog entry, I checked the range of normal shown on my blood tests. In November, 2011, my blood calcium level was 10.0 and the "normal" range listed was 8.0 to 10.0. In September, 2012, my blood calcium level was 10.5 and the normal range was again listed as 8.0 to 10.0. (This 10.5 reading should have triggered a test of my calcium hormone (PTH) level; my doctor also should have brought it my attention.) In October, 2013, when my blood calcium levels were 11.6 and 11.7, the normal range listed was 8.4 to 10.2. The Norman Center would view a calcium level range up to 10.0 as correct on the high end and would disapprove of the 2013 increase to 10.2.

In the words of Dr. Politz, "People don't live with calcium levels 'in the 10s,' no matter what the lab's normal range is. High blood calcium is just not normal." NC blog, 6/5/13. Applying the wrong blood calcium range often contributes to a failure to diagnose excess calcium disease.

At many places on its website, the Norman Center makes the point that the severity of excess calcium disease relates to **duration** of high blood calcium levels, not **how high** the calcium level is. Put another way, a patient with five or six years of blood calcium readings between 10.0 and 10.9 is likely to have suffered more damage than a person with a recent history of blood calcium levels above 11.0. "Organs like the brain, bones, heart and blood vessels, and kidneys are affected by the **duration** of the high blood calcium more than the actual height of the calcium." [emphasis in original] (same blog) Examples follow shortly of serious health consequences resulting from long-term excess calcium disease where the patient never had substantially high blood calcium readings.

Starting at dinner on the cruise ship, Carolyn and I compared blood calcium readings. I can only speak for myself, but I was guilty of trying to one-up her. My assumption was that if my blood calcium reading was higher, then I had a more serious case of excess calcium disease. As I have read more widely, I have learned that the key determinant is the duration of the high blood calcium, not how high the calcium reading is. " . . . [T]he **height of the calcium** (how high it has become) is a very poor predictor of the severity of this disease. It is the **duration** (how long it has been over 10.0) that is associated with all of the complications of high calcium. [emphasis in original] NC blog, 7/11/13.

The Norman Center's blog presents a half-dozen case studies of patients who needed calcium gland surgery and who benefited significantly from it despite having relatively mild levels of high blood calcium. These patients are the subjects of blog entries because they are typical, the rule rather than the exception. **Do not expect your family doctor to be familiar with the modern range for normal blood calcium; expect your PCP to apply too high a "normal range" of blood calcium**. In the words of Dr. Norman, "Since most doctors are not aware that blood calcium levels are different for different ages (heck, we were never taught this either!), they will see your blood calcium level of 10.5 and say 'your calcium is fine . . . it is in the normal range.' If you are over 35, however, nothing could be further from the truth . . . ." (same blog) When my blood calcium level was 10.5 in September, 2012, it was predictable that my doctor would not order a calcium hormone (PTH) test and would fail to tell me that my calcium level was high.

Lisa, age 57, had long duration low-level excess calcium readings of 10.2 to 10.6. Her family doctor labeled them "barely elevated." She was finally referred for surgery after a new doctor ordered a calcium hormone test that yielded high PTH readings of 93 and 97 (versus a normal PTH range of 7 to 53). (My PTH reading in October, 2013 was 127). See NC blog of 6/5/13 by Dr. Politz for more details about Lisa.

Abby, an 83-year-old grandmother from Vermont, had calcium levels between 10.4 and 10.9 for about six years.

She described herself as "a tired, depressed, forgetful, crabby insomniac." Her family thought she was developing Alzheimer's disease. NC blog, 6/7/13 by Dr. Politz.

Phyllis, age 73, had 11 years of high calcium with values ranging from 10.1 to 10.9. The different labs performing her tests used varying scales for "normal" blood calcium. One lab labeled a calcium level of 10.6 as "normal." (This would be true for a teenager, but not an adult.). Given this flawed and misleadingly high "normal" value, her doctor did nothing, noting that her levels were often just barely above the acceptable range. NC blog, 6/21/13 by Dr. Politz.

Cora, age 52, had her blood sent to labs that used "normal range" scales up to 10.6 and even 10.8. As her calcium levels were often within these ranges, " . . . her doctors had absolutely no clue that she had this disease because the lab was providing a normal range for her calcium for ALL humans, not a 52 year old woman!" [emphasis in original] Worse, every time Cora's calcium level went above these artificially high "normal limits," the next year her level would be just within these artificially high limits. Dr. Norman wrote in the Norman Center blog that **"This is a problem we see in about 90% of the charts we review."** [emphasis added] NC blog, 7/11/13. Ultimately Cora's blood was sent to a lab that listed an upper limit of 10.2. This led her to Google and she self-diagnosed with excess calcium disease.

Even medical personnel who are highly knowledgeable about high calcium disease can fail to recognize it. The former chief assistant/nurse to

Dr. Norman, who had become an IT consultant in healthcare, failed to recognize her own symptoms of excess calcium disease. After she received a DEXA bone scan indicating osteopenia (thin bones), she checked her calcium level. She immediately recognized 10.4 as too high, so she had her calcium hormone (PTH) level checked. When it, too, was high, she self-referred to the Norman Center for calcium gland surgery. NC blog, 10/2/13 by Connie Farrell, RN, BSN.

Mrs. S, age 61, had 5 years of calcium readings between 10.0 and 10.9. Her PCP treated her with vitamin D and anti-depressants. After reading about high calcium disease on the Internet, she self-referred to the Norman Center for surgery. Afterwards, Mrs. S returned to her family doctor to communicate her improvement. This led her doctor (Ashok Goyal, MD) to check his own blood calcium level, which had run "between 10.2 and 11.0 for 5 years," but he ignored it because he "knew it was nothing." The post-surgery visit by Mrs. S led this doctor to diagnose excess calcium disease in himself and he, too, had surgery at the Norman Center. NC blog, 10/12/13.

The only three people with high calcium disease I know personally all had blood calcium levels above 11.0. Carolyn's was 11.1; my final levels were 11.6 and 11.7. Walter's blood calcium levels were above 12.0. The seven case histories of patients with mild or only slightly high blood calcium levels make an important point. Recall that the Norman Center sees blood calcium levels that are only slightly above the normal high range "in about 90% of the charts we review." No wonder excess calcium disease is so often not diagnosed.

The Norman Center estimates that 1% of American adults and 2% of American women over age 50 suffer from high calcium disease. As 90% of the medical charts of patients who undergo calcium gland surgery in Tampa reflect only slightly elevated or "mild" high blood calcium, the lesson is clear. Readers need to educate themselves that **in an adult over age 40, a blood calcium reading of 10.0 or above indicates excess calcium disease**.

To learn if you (or a loved one) have excess calcium disease, you need to obtain a copy of your blood test results. Then you should interpret for yourself whether the blood calcium level is high. **You should not rely upon your doctor to decide whether you have high blood calcium**. Too often, a blood calcium level of 10.5 (like my blood calcium level in September, 2012) will be ignored instead of being used to diagnose excess calcium disease.

Dr. Norman is surprisingly gentle when making the point that family doctors cannot be relied upon to recognize what is a high level of blood calcium. He asks readers of the Norman Center blog to educate their treating physicians about what constitutes high blood calcium. In his words, "Most doctors don't understand that calcium levels of 10.2 - 10.6 in an adult over 40 means they have a calcium gland tumor that will make them miserable . . . ." NC blog, 7/11/13.

The Medical Establishment and High Blood Calcium

Dr. Norman's magnanimity about the failure of most PCPs to recognize that a calcium level above 10.0 is "high" is understandable if one consults the conventional wisdom of the medical establishment. For the purposes of this book, the websites of the Mayo Clinic, Harvard Medical School, the National Institute of Health, Wikipedia, and a top rated foreign medical website from the United Kingdom were reviewed at the end of 2014. All five websites were included in the top 10 results of a Google search of "primary hyperparathyroidism." (The New England Journal of Medicine is excluded because it is requires registration and payment.) When a person with high blood calcium searches the Internet for advice, he or she is likely to be directed to these five medical websites (along with the Norman Center website.)

These five websites do not define what is "normal" versus what is "high" blood calcium. However, two sites (Harvard Medical School and Wikipedia) state that surgery to remove a calcium gland tumor is not recommended unless the blood calcium level is 1.0 mg/dl above the normal limit. Thus, if the normal upper limit of blood calcium is defined as 10.0 (Dr. Norman) or 10.2 (my last blood test lab report) or 10.6 (the case study of Phyllis, age 71) or 10.8 (the case study of Cora, age 52), surgery is not recommended unless the blood calcium level is 1.0 higher or above 11.0 or 11.2 or 11.6 or 11.8 using the examples above. Applying this approach, surgery would not have been recommended for any of the case studies from the Norman Center blog described earlier.

Both High Blood Calcium and High PTH Levels?

There are other significant differences between the medical establishment websites and the data presented in the Norman Center blog. These five websites typically state that a diagnosis of excess calcium disease requires **both** a high blood calcium level AND a high PTH level. Yet the introduction to this chapter noted that a "high" calcium hormone level (PTH level) accompanies high blood calcium in only 80% of cases of excess calcium disease. What about the 20% of cases where high blood calcium is not accompanied by a high PTH level?

The source of the 80% figure is the NC blog of 5/9/13, where Dr. Norman wrote: "Our publication in 2010 looking at 10,000 patients with high calcium disease showed that 18% of patients with a large calcium gland tumor (and excess calcium disease) will have all normal calcium hormone [PTH] levels—they don't have a single high PTH level." Again, this data comes from a review of the medical histories of patients who had a calcium gland tumor that was surgically removed, so there is no doubt they had excess calcium disease.

Of the 10,000 surgery patients studied at the Norman Center, the medical history of almost one in five showed no high PTH level. Measurement of the PTH level is not included in routine blood tests; typically it is not measured at all until after a high blood calcium level is reported. Thus, when my first blood test in October, 2013 indicated a very high blood calcium level (11.6), my doctor ordered a second blood calcium test (11.7) together with a calcium hormone (PTH) test. Many of these 10,000 patients were probably like me and had only one calcium hormone (PTH) test. Others, like the case study below, had multiple PTH tests.

Margaret, age 68, had high blood calcium levels (10.5 – 11.0) for at least seven years but also had fluctuating PTH levels in multiple tests. Some were high; some were normal. She was told by her doctor, "You can't have a calcium gland tumor when your calcium hormone (PTH) level is normal. Come on back in six months, but in the meantime take this Fosamax for your [brittle] bones." Elsewhere, Dr. Norman labels such advice as one of the top 10 most common mistakes made by doctors treating patients with excess calcium disease. NC Blog, 8/25/13 (mistake #8). To Dr. Politz, writing about Margaret in the NC blog on 8/28/13: **"Here's the lesson: consistently high blood calcium levels in adults over 35 indicate a calcium gland tumor [and excess calcium disease] almost irrespective of the PTH levels."** [emphasis in original]

At greater length, Dr. Politz explains that in the presence of high blood calcium, even a normal PTH level is abnormally high. The reason is that a healthy calcium gland will regulate the level of calcium hormone in the blood. When the calcium level is too low, the gland secretes calcium hormone (PTH) that leaches calcium from the bones, raising the calcium level in the blood. While this secretion is happening, the PTH level increases. When the calcium level in the blood reaches the desired (normal) level, calcium hormone secretion stops and the PTH level declines. In a patient with high blood calcium, there should be little or no calcium hormone secretion and the PTH level should be low. If a "normal" PTH level accompanies an even mildly high blood calcium level, the PTH level is too high. **"The continued production of calcium hormone (PTH) in the setting of high calcium <u>that should suppress those calcium glands</u> represents autonomous production of calcium hormone (PTH)."** [emphasis in original] This surplus production of calcium hormone (PTH) must be coming from a tumor. NC blog, 8/28/13 by Dr. Politz.

It is not necessary to understand this concept in depth or to attempt to educate one's doctor about the relationship between calcium hormone (PTH) level and blood calcium level. **The presence of a calcium gland tumor and excess calcium disease can be established by a high blood calcium level alone, "irrespective of a high PTH level."** If your doctor does not diagnose or refuses to diagnose high calcium disease because your PTH level is "normal" even though your blood calcium level is high, your doctor is mistaken.

Mainstream Medical Establishment Requirements for High PTH Level

The disparity in how the two "objective" indicators of high calcium disease—high blood calcium and the necessity for high PTH—are treated and when surgery is recommended is shown below.

Mayo Clinic

The Mayo clinic website does not define what constitutes the normal range for blood calcium. It appears to require both high calcium and a high PTH level for a diagnosis, stating " . . . your doctor can make a diagnosis of excess calcium disease if blood tests show you **also** have elevated calcium hormone [PTH]." [emphasis added]

Harvard Medical School

The Harvard Medical School website quotes a 2002 study which recommended surgery only when the blood calcium level is 1.0 above normal and the patient is under age 50. Normal is defined as 10.2 but can vary from lab to lab. However, the Harvard Medical School site also references guidelines published in February, 2009 that acknowledge that surgery might ultimately be recommended because surgery reduces the lifetime risk of fractures. It notes studies indicating that "bone density is likely to start worsening eight to ten years after the diagnosis." Further, "[s]urgery consistently improves bone density and quality of life." The website appears to require both a high calcium and a high PTH level before diagnosis, stating

"Inappropriately high levels of calcium and PTH . . . indicate excess calcium disease."

NIH

The National Institute of Health website (hereafter NIH) states: "Health care providers diagnose excess calcium disease when a person has high blood calcium **and** [high] PTH levels." [emphasis added] The NIH website does not define normal levels of blood calcium and does not list any recommended minimum high calcium level before surgery is recommended.

Wikipedia

Wikipedia states "an elevated level of calcium together with a raised level of calcium hormone [PTH] are typically found" in excess calcium disease. The site quotes the same consensus 2002 recommendations that a patient should be under age 50 and "serum calcium should be 1.0 mg/dl above upper limit of normal" before surgery is indicated. Normal is not defined.

The UK Site

A leading British medical website, patient.co.uk, states the disease is usually diagnosed after blood tests "have shown a high level of calcium **and** a high level of calcium hormone [PTH]." [emphasis added] It does not define the normal range for blood calcium.

Action Items for Readers

1. Always get a copy of your lab test results. Keep them.
2. Check your blood calcium level.
3. Realize your family doctor probably is not familiar with the modern range of normal blood calcium and is likely to apply too high a normal range.
4. Ignore the scale provided in the lab report—it is wrong 75% of the time.
5. Determine for yourself whether your blood calcium level is "high."
6. Remember that a high blood calcium level alone is enough to diagnose excess calcium disease because in 20% of high calcium disease cases, a high PTH level will not be present yet there will still be a calcium gland tumor.
7. Pay $6 and download the Calcium Pro App on-line and enter your blood test results.
8. Be mindful that the longer you have excess calcium disease and the longer you endure high blood calcium, the more damage is done to your body and your mind.

Symptoms—Should I Get a Blood Test?

So far there has been no formal discussion of the symptoms of excess calcium disease. Whether one has the disease is an objective question and the answer is determined by blood test results. But what if there are no recent blood tests to review? What if you have not had a blood test in years? Should you ask your doctor to order a blood test to check for (or eliminate) high calcium disease? Should you leave your doctor out of it and order such a test for yourself? At what cost? To answer these questions, it is useful to review the symptoms of the disease.

Symptoms

At the outset, the reader should be aware that the subject of symptoms of high calcium disease is a source of significant disagreement within the medical community.

On the one hand, the majority of the mainstream medical websites claim in all seriousness that 80% of patients with excess calcium disease are asymptomatic, meaning they have no symptoms at all. The Norman Center, on the other hand, has a list of 21 common symptoms and states that "95% of people with high calcium disease will have 4 or more" and most sufferers will have five or six. In addition, Dr. Norman's shortened description of symptoms is that most patients with excess calcium disease are "miserable" and the disease is robbing them of "the joy of life."

Based on my personal experience and research for this book, I think the Norman Center has the better of this argument by a wide margin. Accordingly, I have taken the Norman Center list and added a few more symptoms from mainstream medical websites to come up with the symptom list below. Exactly how it was derived and special considerations about certain items are discussed later in this chapter.

Excess Calcium Disease Symptom List

1. Chronic fatigue. (#1 symptom) Loss of energy. Don't feel like doing much. Tired all the time and want to nap (but naps don't help).
2. Just don't feel well; don't quite feel normal. Hard to explain but just kind of feel bad.
3. Feel old. Don't have the interest in things that you used to.

4. Can't concentrate, or can't keep concentration like in the past. Worsening memory; forget simple things.
5. Depression.
6. Osteoporosis [bones become brittle and fragile] and Osteopenia [reduced bone mass (less severe than osteoporosis)].
7. Bones hurt, typically in legs and arms.
8. Don't sleep like used to. Wake up in middle of night. Trouble falling asleep.
9. More irritable, harder to get along with, cranky.
10. Gastric acid reflux; heartburn; GERD (gastro esophageal reflux disease).
11. Decrease in sex drive.
12. Thinning hair in middle aged females on front part of scalp.
13. Kidney stones.
14. High blood pressure.
15. Recurrent headaches (patients under 40).
16. Heart palpitations (arrhythmias). Typically atrial arrhythmias.
17. Atrial Fibrillation (rapid heart rate, often requiring thinners and pacemakers).
18. Abnormal liver function tests.
19. Abnormal blood protein levels.
20. Weak and easily tired muscles.
21. Feeling sick (nausea), being sick (vomiting) and feeling off your food.
22. Constipation.
23. Feeling very thirsty and passing urine frequently.
24. Low mood (but not depression).

Now that you have read this list, please heed the following warning. The number one symptom is chronic fatigue. Perhaps the second most common symptoms are low mood and excessive irritability. Almost every time I have described these symptoms, a listener has said, "I hope I have this disease." Most promptly check their blood calcium level (if they have had a recent blood test). To my knowledge, none of my listeners has yet discovered that he or she has excess calcium disease!

Dr. Metchick, an endocrinologist, wrote in the Norman Center blog of 9/18/13 that when he tells a patient that she has high calcium disease, "[t]hese patients are typically very happy to learn that there is a reason they feel bad. They are happy that their problem has a name (excess calcium disease) and they are happy that their problem can be cured with removal of the causative calcium gland tumor."

The normal human desires to have more energy and to be happier may distort your judgment when applying this symptom list to yourself or to someone close to you. This being said, in most parts of the United States, one can order a calcium level blood test without a doctor at a cost of under $30 (see chapter end). There are persons who will read this symptom list, get an inexpensive calcium blood test, learn they have high calcium disease, have surgery to cure it, and thereafter lead a better life. This is why I wrote this book.

History of Symptoms

The medically accepted symptoms of excess calcium disease are changing (though not fast enough to my mind).

According to the Harvard Medical School website: "At one time, the condition was recognized only when it had progressed to the point of causing serious problems such as bone disease, kidney stones, gastrointestinal disorders, and cognitive difficulties." These are the "classic signs and symptoms that clinicians have dubbed '**bones, stones, abdominal moans, and groans.'**" [emphasis added]

Alas, some doctors, including my own, still rely on this old saying. During my 2013 physical, my doctor mentioned learning about "bones, stones, groans, and moans" in medical school. A corollary to this saying, unfortunately, was and sometimes still is that unless a patient has one of these profound symptoms, no diagnosis is made. My PCP told me that although I had high calcium levels in my blood, nothing should be done because my symptoms were not severe enough to justify the risks of surgery to cure the disease. Unfortunately, this was an instance where it was counterproductive to have a doctor as old as I am.

According to Dr. Politz writing in the Norman Center blog of 7/24/13, my doctor's approach is typical. "Some medical doctors still see [calcium gland] surgery the way it was in 1975—big, dangerous, and not very successful." Put another way, your doctor (like mine) may have "learned about high calcium disease from professors who learned from professors who learned from professors back in the dear old 1930s and 40s. They were taught that because this tumor is considered benign, it need not be removed until it makes the patient very sick." (same blog) This approach had some validity "when calcium gland surgery took

4-6 hours and the chance of never talking again after calcium gland surgery was 5-6%." NC blog, 8/25/13. Any perceived validity ended about 1985 and is non-existent in an era of sub-20 minute outpatient calcium gland surgery.

A perfect example of this thinking is the family care physician who diagnosed excess calcium disease in himself only after his patient refused to follow his recommendations for treatment and self-referred herself to the Norman Center for calcium gland surgery. In a 10/12/13 blog entry, Dr. Ashok Goyal, M.D., wrote: " . . . I've diagnosed excess calcium disease a number of times in the past when my patients had really high calcium levels and kidney stones . . . . I thought . . . it isn't much of a problem until the patient gets a broken bone, a kidney stone, or their calcium goes above 12. I also knew that having a calcium gland operation was dangerous . . . [and] avoided sending patients to have [such] surgery until they had one of those problems." He continued: "I knew that calcium gland tumors were not cancerous, the operation was long and tedious, the complications of the operation (when they occurred) were terrible, and so I did nothing for my patients with high blood calcium until they had a kidney stone or broke their leg." In a nutshell, Dr. Goyal (and my doctor) were looking for advanced symptoms reflecting extensive damage caused by high calcium disease.

What explains the disparity between respected medical websites claiming (still) that 80% of persons with excess calcium disease are without any symptoms and the

Norman Center's position, based on over 20,000 surgeries, that almost all sufferers of high calcium disease are "miserable?" The answer lies in the definition of "symptom." Many elements on the Norman Center list are entirely subjective. How does one objectively measure "feel old" or "loss of energy" or "just don't feel well?" Many subjective complaints by themselves or in combination can make patients "feel miserable" without the presence of a single advanced physical symptom.

Norman Center Approach to Symptoms

Let us look more closely at the current list of symptoms from the Norman Center. In slightly abridged form, it reads as follows:

1. Loss of energy. Don't feel like doing much. Tired all the time. Chronic fatigue. (#1 symptom)
2. Just don't feel well; don't quite feel normal. Hard to explain but just kind of feel bad.
3. Feel old. Don't have the interest in things that you used to.
4. Can't concentrate, or can't keep concentration like in the past.
5. Depression.
6. Osteoporosis [bones become brittle and fragile] and Osteopenia [reduced bone mass (less severe than osteoporosis)].
7. Bones hurt, typically in legs and arms.

8. Don't sleep like used to. Wake up in middle of night. Trouble falling asleep.
9. Tired during day and want to nap (but naps don't help).
10. More irritable, harder to get along with, cranky.
11. Worsening memory; forget simple things.
12. Gastric acid reflux; heartburn; GERD (gastro esophageal reflux disease).
13. Decrease in sex drive.
14. Thinning hair in middle aged females on front part of scalp.
15. Kidney stones.
16. High blood pressure.
17. Recurrent headaches (patients under 40).
18. Heart palpitations (arrhythmias). Typically atrial arrhythmias.
19. Atrial Fibrillation (rapid heart rate, often requiring thinners and pacemakers).
20. Abnormal liver function tests.
21. Abnormal blood protein levels.

The Norman Center website says that most people with excess calcium disease "will have 5-6 of these symptoms. Some will have lots of them. A few people will say they don't have any . . . but after an operation they will often say otherwise." In sum, "95% of people with high calcium disease will have 4 or more of these symptoms."

Mainstream Medical Establishment Symptoms

These conclusions are contrary to the views of the mainstream medical establishment. Of the five medical websites reviewed below, three state that 80% of persons with excess calcium disease are without symptoms. (NIH, Harvard, Wikipedia) More and more medical authorities, however, recognize that the subjective complaints on the Norman Center list deserve recognition as symptoms and that family doctors should be screening for them. You, the reader, should screen yourself (or someone close to you) for these often-subjective symptoms.

The Norman Center list of symptoms, while lengthy, is not exhaustive. It does not include one of my most significant symptoms—excess urination.[4] Excess urination is often mentioned as a symptom of high calcium disease on the mainstream medical sites.

The UK Site

Perhaps the second most useful medical website on the subject of symptoms is the UK site, which lists these symptoms:

4 To my layman's understanding, this is a logical symptom. As my bloodstream was flooded with excess calcium, my body took steps to counter the assault. To avoid a buildup of calcium in my kidneys (resulting in painful kidney stones), my body made me thirsty, leading to an large increase in fluid intake and excess urination. When I complained of excess and urgent urination at my 2013 physical, my doctor's recommendation was "drink less water."

- Tiredness
- Weak and easily tired muscles
- Feeling sick (nausea), being sick (vomiting) and feeling off your food
- Constipation
- Tummy (abdominal) pain
- Feeling very thirsty and passing urine frequently
- Depression/low mood

The UK site adds this observation: "You may also have high blood pressure if you have hyperparathyroidism. It is unclear why this happens."[5]

Of the UK site's seven symptoms, two directly relate to the Norman Center list. They are "tiredness" relating to Norman 1, 3, and 9, and "tummy (abdominal) pain" relating to Norman 12 (GERD). Five of the UK site's symptoms do not directly correlate to the experience of the Norman Center. They are "weak and easily tired muscles," food related issues (nausea, vomiting, feeling "off your food"), constipation, feeling very thirsty and passing urine frequently, and low mood (not as severe as depression).

I added these five new or different symptoms from the UK site to the Norman Center list. While I might have been tempted to base these additions on one of my

5 High blood pressure can have many causes and it is unclear if excess calcium disease is one of them, at least according to the mainstream websites. The Norman Center reports that calcium gland surgery often results in a decrease in blood pressure and a reduction in the dosage of blood pressure medications, which can include cessation of such medications. NC blog, 6/23/13.

primary symptoms—excess thirst and urination, a review of the other mainstream websites supports inclusion of all of the UK site's "additional" symptoms.

NIH

The National Institute of Health (NIH) website states boldly that "[m]ost people with excess calcium disease have no symptoms." This statement should be considered controversial and conventional medical wisdom is moving away from this position. As to recognized symptoms, the NIH site is much more similar to the UK site than to the Norman site. Unlike either of these other two sites, however, the NIH breaks symptoms into mild and nonspecific symptoms and more severe symptoms.

In the mild and nonspecific category, the NIH lists muscle weakness (UK), fatigue and increased need for sleep (Norman, 1,9), feelings of depression (Norman 5), and aches and pains in bones (Norman 7) and joints (UK). Under more severe symptoms, the NIH site lists loss of appetite (UK), nausea (UK), vomiting (UK), constipation (UK), confusion or impaired thinking and memory (Norman 4,11) and increased thirst and urination (UK). Ignoring the dichotomy between mild and severe symptoms, the NIH list supports inclusion of all of the UK site's additional symptoms in a comprehensive symptom list.

Mayo Clinic

The Mayo Clinic site does not endorse the position that most people with excess calcium disease have no symptoms.

It states instead that the symptoms of high calcium disease "may be so mild and nonspecific that they don't seem at all related to calcium gland function, or they may be severe." A "mild and nonspecific" symptom is not the same thing as no symptom at all. The Mayo Clinic site appears to endorse subjective complaints as symptoms.

Harvard Medical School

The Harvard Medical School website notes that high calcium disease is "typically discovered in the course of blood testing . . ." and states that about 80% of cases are "asymptomatic (non-symptomatic)." It adds that "there are usually no symptoms or only nonspecific ones, such as fatigue (Norman), constipation (UK), aches and pains (Norman, UK), trouble concentrating (Norman), or low mood (UK)." The Harvard website then adds: "**Excess calcium disease occurs mainly in postmenopausal women, who may blame such vague symptoms on other health problems or just on normal aging.**" [emphasis added]

Wikipedia

Wikipedia states "elevated calcium levels . . . can cause digestive symptoms, kidney stones, mental features and bone disease." Under "signs and symptoms," it repeats the classic formulation of stones, bones, abdominal groans, psychiatric moans, and adds thrones ("refers to polyuria [excessive urination] and constipation").

Wikipedia goes further, however. The Norman Center symptom list reflects its survey of the complaints reported by the more than 20,000 patients who have undergone calcium gland surgery (removal) there. Its symptom list is heavy with subjective symptoms and Norman Center website and blog entries are full of examples of how removal of the calcium gland tumor (and immediate restoration of normal calcium levels) has improved the lives of its patients. Wikipedia begs to differ.

In an entry that appears squarely aimed at the Norman Center's claims, Wikipedia states: "More recently, three randomized controlled trials have studied the role of surgery in patients with asymptomatic excess calcium disease." It then reports that the largest study of the three reported that "[calcium gland] surgery showed increase in bone mass, **but no improvement in quality of life after one to two years . . .**" [emphasis added].

Many comments are appropriate. First, this "largest study" consisted of 191 patients (including 29 men) versus the Norman Center's more than 20,000 patients. Second, the other two of the three studies did show improvement in quality of life after surgery. Third, this book has already quoted the Harvard Medical School website's reference to a February, 2009 study showing that **"Surgery consistently improves bone density and quality of life."** [emphasis added]

Symptoms of Real People

Let us review the symptoms of the three real people I know who have had excess calcium disease. From what I know personally and have been told by Carolyn and Walter about our experiences, the academic review of symptoms presented so far in this chapter needs to be expanded upon.

All three of us mistook our high calcium disease for aging. Nothing more, nothing less. None of us has aged before and we did not know what to expect. All of us are good at "rolling with the punches." But the blows landed by excess calcium disease are not from getting older and the reader should be alert to the possibility that fatigue and low mood are the result of high calcium disease, not simple aging.

Carolyn discovered her high calcium disease as a result of a routine blood test. When she went in for her regular physical, her only significant physical complaints were heavy fatigue and an excessive number of urinary tract infections. When her blood test results showed high calcium and she immediately researched it online, Carolyn quickly recognized the symptoms of excess calcium disease. Bitchiness (her wording), napping on trips to the grocery store (instead of going into the store), inability to complete what had been normal physical activity (walks with Dave)—all resulted from her high calcium disease. And all symptoms immediately disappeared after surgery.

You will learn more about Walter later, but he also attributed any lessening of energy to aging. His particular symptoms related to decreased sensory perceptions (taste, hearing, vision, and smell) and completely escaped his notice. In other words, he was totally unaware of his sensory deficits as opposed to noting them and chalking them up to aging.

Only increased tiredness and lack of energy registered with Walter. As could be expected, he attributed both to getting older. Again, surgery eliminated his symptoms.

An objective record of my "symptoms" was presented in the opening chapter. Overall, I think I did a decent job of communicating my symptoms to my doctor. I knew him well enough to describe the summer of 2013 as "bad" and I am proud of using that description. I mentioned the naps, to no effect, and I brought up excess urination twice, also to no effect. In truth, my recitation of symptoms was essentially irrelevant. As my blood test results with very high blood calcium and PTH levels were the best possible evidence that I had excess calcium disease, my description of symptoms was essentially superfluous.

From a subjective viewpoint, I chalked up how bad I felt to getting older. Like most Americans of retirement age, I was not inclined to look for a physical cause to explain what I felt like; it never really occurred to me to look for anything beyond aging.

For most of my adult life, I have kept a journal. I find it therapeutic to write what is happening and what I am thinking. However, I am not narcissistic enough to go back and reread my journals. Perhaps my children or grandchildren will some day enjoy them or perhaps they will simply make good kindling to start a fire. Only once in a great while, when I need to know the date something happened, will I go back and review one month's journal.

When writing this book, I reviewed two months of the last year before surgery. It was a revelation. I gravitate to people who do not complain about their physical ailments (or anything else); I prefer people who can take the bad with the good. As I reviewed two months of journal entries, though, I could see evidence of excess calcium disease everywhere.

The best example is GERD or gastro-intestinal reflux disease. In laymen's terms, this medical condition refers to stomach acid coming up from the stomach into the esophagus. According to Wikipedia, symptoms include heartburn, regurgitation and nausea. I did not mention GERD at my physical and it never occurred to me that I suffered from it. However, when I reread the journals from January and February 2013, 12 months before surgery, I found myself suffering from stomach upsets several times a week. I always attributed this to diet or something I had eaten. No connection to GERD came to mind.

Example two is poor physical conditioning and my resulting frustration. Like most people, I view one's physical conditioning as a matter of personal responsibility. If one is fat and out of shape, it is one's own fault. (This approach is reflected in the journal entries surrounding my doctor visit in the fall of 2013.) Early in 2013, I wrote "As I walked this morning, I thought to myself "this exercise regime is fit for an 80 year old man, not a 65 year old. When am I going to step it up?" I was often hard on myself, entreating myself to exercise more, lose weight, cheer up. On February 6,

I wrote, "No walk this morning. It is not just laziness. It is more that I would be out of action for several hours [from fatigue caused by walking]. No, it is mostly laziness." In retrospect, I am relieved that it was not laziness, but something with a physical cause.

The most graphic example of my frame of mind is in the journal entry of Saturday, February 16, 2013, where I wrote: "Which brings me to a bigger topic. A 40-minute walk along the beach is not sufficient exercise for me at age 65. Maybe at age 85. But not now." I continued: "When I look at myself in the mirror, I see no muscle tone. Indeed, almost no muscles at all in my upper body. As I starve myself down from [my present weight], I become skin and bone and rolls of fat. I have to add muscle work. Maybe, just maybe, [at my San Juan Islands home] I can carry wood, shovel, and do other manual labor for some muscle workouts." But physical work never happened in the summer of 2013. I blamed myself for this sloth, this lack of exercise and work. As it turned out, there was a physical explanation for my lack of conditioning and strength, but I was unaware of it and blamed myself instead.

Enough. The point is that you, the reader, may be completely unaware of your symptoms. If you have high blood calcium and excess calcium disease, it is likely you will look back after surgery and see all the symptoms you missed. It happened with Carolyn and with Walter and with me. The symptoms are there. You simply do not see them. And, most likely, you are blaming yourself for the condition you are in, to the detriment of your mental health and happiness.

Recommendation—Get a Blood Test

The modern trend is to recognize subjective complaints as symptoms and not to refer to patients with no advanced or objective symptoms as "asymptomatic." The Harvard Medical School site acknowledges that "some experts consider 'asymptomatic' something of a misnomer because of the many nonspecific complaints associated with the disease. However, . . . people often discount them and don't seek medical attention for them." This is an important point. Just because you, the reader (or someone close to you), may be so accustomed to your subjective complaints that you have not sought medical treatment, these subjective symptoms may still indicate the presence of excess calcium disease. At the least, they may be cause to get a blood test to learn your blood calcium level.

So let us adopt this approach. If you have even an inkling that there may a physical explanation for how bad you feel, end the suspense. Get a blood test.

Can I get a calcium blood test without a doctor? Cost?

Yes. Under $30.

One can pay a lot for a calcium blood test. It is included in routine blood tests that can cost between $283 and $675 according to the website health.costhelper.com. An August 2011 article on calcium tests at the website medicalnewstoday.com ended by stating that calcium tests "can cost up to $500" and the cost may not be paid by insurance.

It is possible to go on-line to order much cheaper blood tests for yourself. A mid-January, 2015 visit to the website walkinlab.com ["Walk-In-Lab"] yielded the following information. A blood test to measure blood calcium level (not PTH level) cost $29. Or for $27 one could order what is called a Comprehensive Metabolic Panel (CMP-14), which includes calcium level. It is "a group of 14 laboratory tests . . . to give information about the current status of your liver, kidneys, and electrolyte and acid/base balance [and] blood sugar and blood proteins . . . ." A calcium test is also included in a Basic Metabolic Panel, which costs $26 at Walk-In-Lab as BMP8, a group of 8 tests.

Note: **Do not order** the more expensive PTH level test ($159). Unless your blood calcium level is above normal, there is no need to order a PTH test. If your calcium level is high and you then choose to order the PTH test as a follow-up, remember that in 20% of cases of excess calcium disease, the PTH level is normal even when the calcium level is high. Thus, a normal PTH level does not rule out high calcium disease.

The Walk-In-Lab website says no doctor is necessary. A telephone call to the 800 number of Walk-In-Lab confirms this. Just go on-line, pick your test, print out your order, and take it to the nearest lab of your choice as shown on the website. No doctor need be involved.

Action Items for Readers

1. Review the list of 24 symptoms early in this chapter. How many apply to you or to someone close to you?
2. Also review Dr. Norman's shorter description of how a person with excess calcium disease feels ("miserable" and missing "the joy of life"). Does this apply to you or to someone close to you?
3. Be aware that a normal desire to have more energy and to be happier may distort your judgment.
4. If you have any inkling that you (or someone close to you) may have excess calcium disease, GET A CALCIUM LEVEL BLOOD TEST! No doctor is needed and there is much to gain and little to lose beyond the cost of the test (under $30).
5. Do not get the more expensive PTH level blood test unless your calcium level is high.

Monitoring or Surgery?

Okay, you have excess calcium disease. You know this because your blood calcium is above the normal range, a range you applied yourself (above 10.0). Perhaps you obtained a (costly) PTH test as well. If it is high, it is confirmation of the presence of high calcium disease. If the PTH level is normal, in all likelihood you may still have excess calcium disease because in 20% of cases, high blood calcium is not accompanied by a high PTH level.

You know you have high calcium disease. Does your doctor? Do you care if your doctor does not correctly diagnose the disease? The answer may surprise you.

The split in recognition of symptoms (or how symptoms are defined by the mainstream medical establishment, on the one hand, and the Norman Center, on the other) is important here. As we have seen, three of the five "conventional wisdom" medical websites state that 80% of persons with excess calcium disease are asymptomatic—they have no symptoms. The Norman Center doctors disagree strongly; the Center's website lists 21 symptoms, most of which are subjective.

The medical establishment recommends that most persons with "asymptomatic" excess calcium disease should be **monitored**. Period. No surgery. The Norman Center, composed of four surgeons who perform up to 12 calcium gland surgeries a day, begs to differ. It seems safe to conclude that the Norman Center believes that essentially all persons with high calcium disease should have surgery as soon as possible to cure the disease once and for all. In a blog entry dated 6/23/13, Dr. Norman wrote: "We now perform an average of 52 calcium gland surgeries weekly on patients from all over the world." He continues, "[E]very day we see patients treated by doctors who have no clue about the high risks of "watching" the high blood calcium, thinking that 'since the calcium is not that high, we can just keep checking it to see if it goes higher." According to Dr. Norman, "It takes 20 minutes (often less) to cure almost all patients of high calcium disease, leading to tremendous health benefits for the rest of your life." (same blog)

The decision of whether to monitor the disease or to undergo surgery to cure it is for you to make, not your doctor. Recall that because excess calcium disease is an objective condition, health insurance and Medicare will pay for surgery to cure it (by removing the calcium gland tumor) without any referral from a doctor. To assist in your decision, let us further examine the rationale for each position.

Mainstream Medical Websites and Monitoring

Mayo Clinic

The Mayo Clinic website contains a section titled "**Watchful waiting.**" The site explains: "Your doctor may recommend no treatment [for high calcium disease] and regular monitoring if:

- Your calcium levels are only slightly elevated
- Your kidneys are functioning normally, and you have no kidney stones
- Your bone density is normal or only slightly below normal
- You have no other symptoms that may improve with treatment"

According to the Mayo Clinic, "[i]f you choose this watch-and-wait approach, you'll likely need periodically scheduled tests to monitor your blood-calcium levels and bone density." The Mayo Clinic website suggests that if you are to be monitored, you should watch how much calcium and vitamin D is in your diet. As discussed later, the Norman Center blog establishes unequivocally that Vitamin D supplements and foods high (or low) in calcium have nothing to do with high calcium disease or its treatment.

Acknowledging that surgery "is the most common treatment for excess calcium disease and provides a cure in about 95% of all cases," the Mayo Clinic site states that "[s]urgery may be done as an outpatient procedure, allowing you to go home the same day. In such cases, the surgery can be done through very small incisions in the neck, and you receive only local anesthetics." Note the use of plural "incisions" here; the Norman Center surgeons make one small one-inch incision in the front of the neck, not multiple small incisions.

NIH

While the NIH website recognizes that "[s]urgery to remove the overactive calcium gland or glands is the only definitive treatment for excess calcium disease . . .," the NIH also endorses monitoring. Its website states: "Some people who have mild excess calcium disease may not need immediate or even any surgery and **can be safely monitored.**" [emphasis added] Such "[p]eople may wish to talk with their health care provider about long-term monitoring if they "are symptom-free" [and] "have only slightly elevated blood calcium levels [and] have normal kidneys and bone density." Further, "[l]ong term monitoring should include periodic clinical evaluations, annual [blood calcium] measurements, annual [checks of kidney function], and bone density measurements every 1 to 2 years." When reading these extensive recommendations, it is useful to realize that the cost of monitoring may exceed the cost of surgery.

The NIH site recognizes that "[e]ating, diet, and nutrition have **not** been shown to play a role in causing or preventing excess calcium disease." [emphasis added] It adds that "[p]eople with high calcium disease without symptoms who are being monitored do not need to restrict calcium in their diets." However, the NIH site also states that **"Vitamin D deficiency should be corrected if present."** [emphasis added] It continues: "Experts suggest correcting vitamin D deficiency in people with excess calcium disease . . ." and "Research is ongoing to determine optimal doses and regimes of vitamin D supplementation for people with high calcium disease." Then, apropos of nothing, the NIH site lists the guidelines for vitamin D consumption "for the healthy public."

The Norman Center believes that low Vitamin D confuses about 50% of endocrinologists. NC blog, 8/25/13. The Norman Center website and blog entries establish that Vitamin D consumption has nothing to do with mitigating or curing excess calcium disease. While patients with excess calcium disease typically have low levels of Vitamin D, "over 95% of people with a calcium gland tumor (and excess calcium disease) will have low vitamin D." And "the older the tumor, the lower the vitamin D . . . ." NC blog, 9/18/13 by Dr. Metchick, an endocrinologist.

Perhaps the endocrinologists think the calcium gland(s) are over-active and provide too much calcium hormone (PTH) because the patient has a low vitamin D level. No! The calcium gland(s) are overactive because there is a tumor (or tumors)! "There is no mechanism by which a low vitamin D can result in high blood calcium (vitamin D is required by humans to absorb calcium from the foods we eat)." NC blog, 8/25/13. "You cannot give Vitamin D to a person with high blood calcium—it will make the calcium go higher. NC blog, 5/30/13.

Let us expand upon this point. If "vitamin D is required by humans to absorb calcium from the foods we eat," it follows that a person low in Vitamin D would not (or may not) be absorbing enough calcium from her food. The result would be too little calcium in the blood, the opposite condition of high calcium disease. Increasing the vitamin D level (by using Vitamin D supplements, for example) would increase calcium absorption from food being consumed. This should increase blood calcium levels. Why would any doctor prescribe Vitamin D supplements, intended to result in higher blood calcium levels, to a person with high calcium disease who, by definition, already has elevated blood calcium? A better outcome is to surgically remove the calcium gland tumor (or tumors) causing the excessive secretion of calcium hormone (PTH).

Since giving Vitamin D to a person with high calcium disease will make his or her blood calcium level go even higher, it is astonishing that mainstream medical websites like the NIH site suggest Vitamin D supplements. It is no wonder that 50% of endocrinologists are confused about Vitamin D and that so many doctors prescribe Vitamin D supplements that are useless or counterproductive.

Wikipedia

Wikipedia has such an extreme position regarding surgery that an endorsement of monitoring must be implied. Again, the site quotes a 2002 study containing recommendations that surgery is not appropriate for high calcium disease unless patients are under age 50 and have calcium levels at least 1.0 above "normal."

Harvard Medical School

Harvard Medical School's website recommends surgery when excess calcium disease "causes severe symptoms," but otherwise recommends monitoring. The Harvard website observes that patients progress from asymptomatic to "a more serious condition" about one third of the time. Recognizing this, "some experts favor simply monitoring most patients and, if necessary, managing the condition with lifestyle measures and medications." But **the Harvard site also recognizes that other experts argue that the cost of monitoring may exceed the cost of calcium gland surgery.** It acknowledges that surgery eliminates any risk of disease progression and may also get rid of many subjective complaints.

The Harvard site references guidelines published in the February, 2009 issue of *The Journal of Clinical Endocrinology and Metabolism* in which experts **"determined that surgery might ultimately be recommended even for the most asymptomatic patients"** because surgery reduces the lifetime risk of fractures. The Harvard Medical School website recognizes that studies indicate that **"bone density starts worsening 8 to 10 years after the diagnosis"** and **"[s]urgery consistently improves bone density and quality of life."** [emphasis added]

UK site

The UK website squarely presents the split of opinions on surgery versus monitoring. It states: "If you have mild excess calcium disease with a mildly raised calcium level and little in the way of symptoms, your doctor may just suggest that you be regularly monitored." This usually includes blood tests to check on calcium levels and kidney function, regular blood pressure checks, and monitoring of your symptoms. [It] can include DEXA bone scanning. Unlike the four American medical websites, the UK site explicitly acknowledges that **"this monitoring approach is considered controversial by some"** [emphasis added] and recommends discussing the pros and cons with your doctor.

The Norman Center

As reflected in numerous blog entries, the surgeons at the Norman Center see no advantage and many disadvantages to monitoring patients with high calcium disease. The Center's website repeatedly makes the point that it is the duration of the disease, not the level of calcium in the blood, that determines the damage caused by the disease.

Dr. Politz phrases it this way: "The lesson here is simple. Calcium gland tumors are not harmless even though they are technically benign. If you see what they do to patients over the course of years, you would conclude that they are not so benign in the way that they act." NC blog, 6/21/13 by Dr. Politz. He continues, "Calcium gland tumors will slowly strip away the health of one organ at a time—just like many cancers do. Excess calcium disease can be entirely cured by removing the tumor . . . ." He concludes, "We can't fall into the trap of thinking the patient can just live with high calcium disease just because the calcium is 'just a little bit high.' If you live with it; you'll die with it. Simple as that." (same blog)

Two case studies deserve mention here. Jane, a 56 year old from Orlando, Florida was seen at the Norman Center with stage 4 kidney failure. She had untreated excess calcium disease for more than a decade. Her nephrologist, or kidney specialist, had treated her with high dose Vitamin D. The Norman Center blog on 5/30/13 labeled this medical care "ignorant," adding that if you give Vitamin D to a person with high blood calcium, "it will make the calcium go higher." Jane would not have had stage 4 kidney failure if calcium gland surgery had been performed as early as possible.

After discussing a frightful and rare case of a teenager with high calcium disease who was "monitored" by his doctors, Dr. Norman wrote: "[P]lease, remember, excess calcium disease is not to be 'monitored.' These [calcium gland] tumors destroy the body in ALL patients, so waiting for something bad to occur is dumb." [emphasis in original] NC blog, 5/9/13.

Surgery? What kind of surgery?

The five mainstream medical websites present two surgical options. In addition, the Norman Center has developed a fast out-patient surgery in which a patient typically has a one inch incision in the neck, followed by a check of all four calcium glands during which the health of each gland is checked in real-time. Calcium glands with tumors are removed; those that remain have been confirmed to be healthy. This surgery usually takes under 20 minutes and patients are released within 90 minutes to three hours.

The mainstream medical websites do not contain a description of the Norman Center's calcium gland surgery. Usually these medical websites divide surgery into two versions described on the Harvard Medical School site as follows: "The standard surgery, called bilateral neck exploration, entails making a two- to five- inch incision across the front of the neck, examining all four calcium glands, and removing the enlarged ones. It's usually performed under general anesthesia . . . ." There is also "minimally invasive surgery . . . [which] involves a smaller, one- to two- inch incision, takes less time, and requires less anesthesia. **"This technique can be used whenever preoperative imaging indicates there is a single abnormal calcium gland."** [emphasis added]

The Norman Center doctors would object that this is not the surgery they perform. Calcium gland surgery at the Norman Center (as I understand it) checks all four calcium glands (like a "bilateral neck surgery"), removes all calcium gland tumors (not just "a single tumor"), and does not rely upon preoperative imagery to locate tumors.

The Mayo Clinic site makes reference to outpatient surgery but, as seen, refers to multiple incisions for minimally invasive surgery.

The NIH site describes two kinds of surgery but uses different names as follows: "Standard neck exploration 'involves a larger incision that allows the surgeon to access and examine all four calcium glands and remove the overactive ones [those with a tumor]. This type of surgery is more extensive and typically requires a hospital stay of 1 to 2 days. Surgeons use this approach if they plan to inspect more than one gland.'" Minimally invasive calcium gland surgery "may be used when only one of the calcium glands is likely to be overactive [have a tumor]. **Guided by [the preoperative scan], the surgeon makes a small incision in the neck to remove the gland."** . . . [P]atients typically have less pain and a quicker recovery than with more invasive surgery." [emphasis added] The Norman Center surgeons would distance their operation from this description, too, because they do not use preoperative scans to locate calcium gland tumors. Indeed, the Norman Center blog repeatedly warns against this practice.

Neither Wikipedia nor the UK site discusses different types of calcium gland surgery.

What if your doctor does diagnose the disease?

Let us return to the question asked at the beginning of this chapter. If you know you have high calcium disease, should you care whether your doctor diagnoses it?

You may be better off if your doctor, like mine, misses the diagnosis. The reason is that your doctor may recommend or implement monitoring of your excess calcium disease without ever telling you that you have it. This can happen several ways. My doctor de facto implemented monitoring by telling me that "there is nothing worth doing" with respect to my high blood calcium.

There was no acknowledgment of the disease or of a tumor on the calcium gland or of low risk surgery as a viable option to remove the tumor. We talked for a minute or two and then moved along with only the suggestion that I drink less water.

Many PCPs, having made a diagnosis of high calcium disease, would refer you to an endocrinologist. Recall that when I quizzed my new doctor at an HMO-like organization, he answered that all he knew about high blood calcium was that if it appeared, he was to refer the patient to an endocrinologist.

Whether you should accept a referral to an endocrinologist and what the endocrinologist may do is the subject of the next chapter. A shortened version is this. The endocrinologist may implement monitoring. Even if the endocrinologist recommends surgery, he or she may order imaging tests such as sestamibi scans or ultrasound that greatly delay the calcium gland surgery. According to the Norman Center blog, when sestamibi scans are ordered, surgery is delayed by 3 months to two and a half years on average. Given the risk that this specialist may recommend or implement monitoring (without ever giving you the choice) or conduct expensive pre-surgery tests that delay calcium gland surgery, you should seriously consider refusing a referral to an endocrinologist.

Action Items for Readers

1. Many doctors will not recognize or diagnose excess calcium disease until it becomes severe and manifests serious objective symptoms (bones, stones, moans, and groans).
2. If you know you have excess calcium disease and your doctor does anything other than recommend immediate calcium gland surgery, you are being monitored (without your permission).
3. The only cure for high calcium disease is calcium gland surgery. The descriptions of calcium gland surgery in the mainstream medical websites are outdated and misleading. Compare the description of surgery at the Norman Center (and the video (under 20 minutes)).
4. The costs of monitoring excess calcium disease can exceed the cost of surgery.
5. Remember the severity of high calcium disease correlates to the duration of the disease (how long you have had it), not the level of calcium in your blood. The longer you have untreated excess calcium disease, the more damage it does to your body and your mind.
6. Refuse any Vitamin D supplements; more Vitamin D will not mitigate or cure high calcium disease and may be counterproductive.
7. Read the next chapter before deciding whether to accept a referral to an endocrinologist.

Should I See an Endocrinologist?

It should be apparent by now that most PCPs or family doctors are not knowledgeable about excess calcium disease. In one of the very first entries in the Norman Center's blog, Dr. Norman wrote: " . . . [m]any doctors are not quite up to date about high blood calcium and excess calcium disease." NC blog, 5/9/13. Before the end of the blog's first month, this had escalated to "If you are reading this [blog entry], it is very likely that you know more about excess calcium disease than your doctor does." NC blog, 5/30/13.

In part because of widespread unfamiliarity with excess calcium disease, referrals are common. (Option B is that your doctor is so clueless about the disease that no referral is made. My doctor was in this category.) If you belong to an HMO or go to an HMO-like organization, your high blood calcium is likely to lead to a referral, regardless of whether excess calcium disease has been diagnosed.

What type of doctor will you be referred to? Most likely, it will be an endocrinologist. The website hormone.org defines endocrinologists as "specially trained physicians who diagnose diseases related to the glands. The diseases they are trained to treat often affect other parts of the body beyond glands. While primary care doctors know a lot about the human body, for diseases and conditions directly related to glands they will usually send a patient to an endocrinologist." The website adds, "The glands in a person's body release hormones. Endocrinologists treat people who suffer from hormonal imbalances . . . ." A list of eleven common conditions treated by endocrinologists follows; it does not include high calcium disease but does include osteoporosis [brittle bones] that can result from excess calcium disease.

By this point, you should know whether you have excess calcium disease. Using your blood calcium level, you can make this diagnosis just as knowledgeably as your doctor. (By analogy to the Norman blog entry quoted above, if you have read this far, you probably know far more about excess calcium disease than does your doctor.) Given that you know you have the disease, you should seriously contemplate refusing any referral to an endocrinologist. This chapter will explain why you may decide not to see an endocrinologist at all.

The Endocrinologist's Employment Disease

When President Bush signed a new estate tax law on June 7, 2001, its complicated nature led BusinessWeek to refer to it in the next issue as "The Accountants Employment Act." In similar fashion, high calcium disease could be referred to as "The Endocrinologist's Employment Disease."

Endocrinologists can be "fully employed" by excess calcium disease only by monitoring and/or testing it. When you are first seen, it is highly likely the endocrinologist will order substantial testing, which amounts to monitoring. In this context, anything other than surgery to remove the calcium gland tumor amounts to monitoring.

The mainstream medical websites contain lengthy descriptions of tests likely to be ordered by an endocrinologist. It is not necessary to repeat those descriptions here. Suffice to say that the Mayo Clinic and the NIH websites describe a bone mineral density test (DXA scan) to check for brittle bones, urine tests (24 hour collection of urine) to check kidney function, CT scans of your abdomen to check for kidney stones, and ultrasound tests (same). The NIH site also suggests a "25-hydroxy-vitamin D blood test" to check your Vitamin D level.

None of these tests cure anything. Nor do they help diagnose high calcium disease (the blood test result establishes that.) Rather they measure how much damage the untreated calcium gland tumor has done to your body so far. After reviewing these test results, the endocrinologist will decide between "Watchful waiting" (Mayo Clinic website) and a referral to a surgeon.

If you challenge an endocrinologist about the necessity for or utility of undergoing these tests, he or she will likely explain that the tests are the normal, recommended course of treatment for persons with high calcium disease.

A survey of the mainstream medical websites supports this view. These costly, time-consuming, and non-curative tests are explained and, by implication, recommended by the UK site and the websites of Harvard Medical School, the Mayo Clinic, and the NIH. (Wikipedia refers to medical imaging and to other testing). Your endocrinologist may never have encountered resistance or refusal to undergo the recommended testing. Stick to your guns!

The view of the Norman Center surgeons is that this testing (monitoring) is unnecessary and can be counterproductive. Yet the mainstream medical websites list and define all these tests at length because they are in common use. If you accept a referral to an endocrinologist, you should anticipate being subjected to the time and expense involved in undergoing this testing. The results will not be of material assistance in deciding whether you have the disease (you know this already) or what course of treatment to pursue. But the tests will keep the endocrinologist fully employed with your case for quite some time. You, the reader, should realize that you do not have to consent to any testing and that if you do, it may significantly delay curing your disease because it will postpone surgery.

My reading of the Norman Center website and Dr. Norman's biography on the Center's blog leads to the conclusion that he is both a surgeon and an endocrinologist. The doctor is not fond of his fellow endocrinologists.

In the blog entry of 7/3/13, Dr. Norman wrote: "Most endocrinologists are not very good at excess calcium disease." Continuing on, he tells patients to "stop going to endocrinologists who do dumb things . . . . If you could see the nonsense we see every single day . . . ." The Norman Center blog provides ample evidence to prove his point.

Dumb things #1 and #2 are probably recommending the standard tests described above and then recommending the monitoring of your excess calcium disease (with or without Vitamin D supplements). Nothing more needs to be added on these subjects.

Sestamibi Scans

Dumb thing #3 is the use of sestamibi scans. Not overuse, but any use. The Mayo Clinic explains a sestamibi scan as follows: "Sestamibi is a radioactive compound that is absorbed by overactive calcium glands and can be detected by a scanner that detects radioactivity. The normal thyroid gland also absorbs sestamibi. To eliminate uptake in the thyroid obscuring the uptake in a calcium tumor, radioactive iodine, which is only taken up by the thyroid, is also given and the thyroid image is digitally subtracted."

Got that? In layman's language, the patient is given a radioactive compound that is absorbed by a calcium gland tumor (but not by a healthy calcium gland) and also by the thyroid. The patient also is given radioactive iodine, which is absorbed by the thyroid but not by the calcium gland tumor (or by a healthy calcium gland). The image of the thyroid, shown by the radioactive iodine, is digitally removed (think Photoshop!) leaving only the calcium gland tumor visible.

Does this work? Nope. Or at least not very well. What the Mayo Clinic does not state explicitly is that sestamibi scans are typically fuzzy, out of focus, hard-to-read black and white x-ray-like sheets.

When Carolyn, my cruise dinner friend, was about to go into surgery, her surgeons and a lab technician poured over her sestamibi scan (?) or MRI (?) in her presence to try to locate her calcium gland tumor. Carolyn says that the surgery would have gone ahead even if the tumor was not located, but one wonders. When she told me about the surgery, she said that the technician present, who had the most experience in reading these scans, pointed to a dark, fuzzy area and said "I think that's it!" Based on this "reading" of the scan, Carolyn's surgery went ahead.

According to Norman Center data as presented in its blog, sestamibi scans are wrong 100% of the time when they are negative (showing no calcium gland tumor) and 60% of the time when positive (showing such a tumor.) NC blog, 7/3/13. The scans are accurate only 20% of the time when locating small calcium gland tumors and, as discussed below, they never show more than one tumor. NC blog, 6/8/13.

According to Dr. Norman, "[Sestamibi] scans are emphasized by insecure surgeons and inexperienced endocrinologists." (same blog) The problem is that very few surgeons do a lot of calcium gland surgeries. Surgeons are rightfully "insecure." These inexperienced surgeons attempt to use a sestamibi scan to locate the calcium gland tumor—to determine which of the four calcium glands has a tumor—before surgery begins. If the scan is negative (does not show any calcium gland tumor), often these surgeons will not operate at all. Period.

Be aware that these "insecure surgeons" are following the recommended surgical procedure described in the mainstream medical websites for minimally invasive surgery. See websites of Harvard Medical School, Mayo Clinic, and NIH. The surgical procedure to first find the tumor (by preoperative imaging) and only then to operate is soundly criticized by the Norman Center surgeons.

According to the Norman Center, a negative scan of a patient with high blood calcium (and excess calcium disease) is wrong 100% of the time. The high blood calcium proves that there is a calcium gland tumor—it is always there. A negative scan does not mean that the tumor is not there; it simply means the tumor did not show up. Often it is hidden behind the nearby thyroid gland. Even when a sestamibi scan shows a calcium gland tumor, Norman Center data indicates that the location shown is wrong 60% of the time. NC blog, 7/3/13.

Recall that up to 30% of persons with high calcium disease have more than one calcium gland tumor. Sestamibi scans never show the presence of multiple calcium gland tumors. "Scans almost never show two tumors when they are present—they only show one (or zero)." NC blog, 6/8/13. As discussed later, all tumors must be removed before the disease is cured.

The Norman Center recommends that patients not have a sestamibi scan at all before coming to Tampa for surgery. This applies to self-referred patients, like me, and to referrals from doctors as well.

Ectopic Glands

The Norman Center does use sestamibi scans and I had one in Tampa before my surgery. (See next chapter.) The purpose of the scan was not to locate my calcium gland tumor, which the doctors knew was there, but to locate what are known as ectopic calcium glands.

Most calcium glands are located near the thyroid gland. Hence their medical name of "parathyroid" glands (about or near the thyroid). Ectopic calcium glands are not located near the thyroid. "If they are up under the jaw or down into the chest we call them 'ectopic calcium glands.'" NC blog, 8/5/13. This is not a problem "as long as your surgeon recognizes it *prior* to your operation, and knows anatomy and embryology enough to know how to find [calcium gland tumors] (without digging around in your neck for a dozen hours!)." [emphasis in original] (same blog)

The Norman clinic uses sestamibi scans for the limited purpose of locating ectopic calcium glands, which are present in 5% of patients. **"We PREFER negative scans!"** [emphasis in original] NC blog, 6/8/13. "If the scan is negative, we are happy as clams, knowing that the patient does not have an ectopic calcium gland and their calcium gland tumor is 'para' (around) the thyroid gland." (same blog) What if the scan is positive? "ALL other doctors (and all patients!) want to see a positive scan. WE DO NOT. We do the exact same operation on ALL people and **having a positive scan does not save us even 10 seconds in the operating room.**" [emphasis in original] (same blog)

Dr. Norman has written that he is one of the inventors and developers of many of the techniques used for sestamibi scans. " . . . I can tell you that these scans are not reliable enough to be used to make ANY decisions about your health . . . whether you should have excess calcium gland surgery or not, what operation to have, or how many bad calcium glands will be found. Scans can't tell this information! Scans are overemphasized and CANNOT be used to make any decisions!" [emphasis in original] NC blog, 6/8/13.

Other Imaging Tests

Endocrinologists and surgeons also order ultrasound and CT scans in connection with calcium gland surgery. Dr. Norman is just as frustrated by their use. In his view, "sestamibi scans, ultrasound, and CT scans . . . are not good enough to tell who has one calcium gland tumor and who has more than one. Excess calcium disease surgery relying on these imaging tests is a bad trend." (same blog)

Robert, from Boston, was subjected to numerous unsuccessful imaging tests that delayed his surgery for years. His family doctor, fed up with delays attributed to negative scan results, finally sent Robert to Tampa because the endocrinologist was "doing nothing because he couldn't find the tumor with his ultrasound machine!" NC blog, 7/3/13. Robert's history included 21 high blood calcium levels, 16 high PTH levels, bad osteoporosis [brittle bones], 3 bouts of kidney stones, and some kidney failure.

"[Robert was] literally dying of high calcium disease but his endocrinologist ('an expert at a major Boston university' ????) never sent him to a surgeon because he can't find the calcium gland tumor on ultrasound . . . . Robert had 2 sestamibi scans and 7 ultrasound scans over 5.5 years and was allowed to suffer for no reason." His surgery took 8 minutes. Dr. Norman wrote: **"The absurdity of a man dying of a [calcium gland] tumor that takes 8 minutes to cure is beyond comprehension."** [emphasis added] (same blog)

The Norman Center blog entry of 5/21/13 discusses a 72-year-old man who had high blood calcium for 11 years with 4 high PTH levels. His surgeons in Syracuse declined to operate because of a negative sestamibi scan. A woman with a blood calcium reading of 11.6 (identical to mine) but a negative sestamibi scan was denied surgery by her doctors because "nothing could be done." Instead, they started her on Vitamin D, which caused her calcium to go even higher. NC blog, 9/18/13 by Dr. Metchick.

Be aware that getting a sestamibi scan will always delay surgery. According to the Norman Center blog, "When endocrinologists get a sestamibi scan they delay calcium gland surgery by 3 months to 2.9 years. If the scan is positive it delays surgery by nearly 3 months. If the scan is negative it delays surgery by almost 3 years." NC blog, 8/25/13.

Dr. Metchik, the endocrinologist who wrote a guest blog on 9/18/13, no longer performs sestamibi scans. He simply refers his patients to the Norman Center.

Never Undergo a Needle Biopsy of Your Calcium Gland Tumor

One of the most dangerous things an endocrinologist can do is to perform a needle biopsy of a calcium gland tumor. Yet a mainstream medical website, the UK site, lists a needle biopsy as one of the "further investigations" a patient should expect (and endure). The UK website states: "A biopsy of one of your calcium glands may be suggested. This is a sample that is taken from the gland, using a needle. It is usually carried out using scanning, such as ultrasound, to guide the doctor who is taking the biopsy. A biopsy may help to exclude [cancer]." As calcium gland tumors are almost never cancerous, this risk is too low to merit a needle biopsy.

Calcium gland tumor cells will grow anywhere. "These are not cancerous cells, but if you drop a piece of the calcium gland tumor into the neck during an operation [or a needle biopsy] then these cells will start growing." The Norman Center blog reported eleven patients from all over the U.S. with this problem. "These patients are VERY hard to cure, and almost all of them require multiple operations every year or two so we can remove the new weeds (calcium gland tumor implants) that grew. NC blog, 8/14/13.

Recommendations

Dr. Norman urges patients (and I urge people reading this book) to "please educate yourself and don't let your doctor do dumb things because they can't find the tumor on a scan . . . . NC blog, 7/3/13. I make a broader recommendation. The best way to keep your doctor from doing dumb things or from delaying surgery and a cure is "Avoid endocrinologists!"

Action Items for Readers

1. If you are referred to an endocrinologist, ask why! Remember that you can refuse the referral. Even if your doctor and the endocrinologist are genuinely offended or puzzled by your refusal, do not feel guilty. It is likely to save you money and to speed up your surgery and cure.
2. If you know you have excess calcium disease, question why it is necessary to undergo any testing (with associated expense and delay) before having surgery to cure the disease.
3. Never allow your endocrinologist or any doctor to perform a needle biopsy of your calcium gland tumor. The tumor is not cancerous and the procedure is dangerous!
4. If any costs of testing will be paid directly by you (entire cost not covered by health insurance or Medicare), just say no!
5. If a sestamibi scan or other imaging test is suggested, ask whether the result will affect whether surgery goes forward and how soon the surgery will happen. You can refuse to consent to a sestamibi scan. Be certain you understand why the scan is being performed before consenting.
6. If you are certain you have excess calcium disease, consider an immediate self-referral to the Norman Center in Tampa, Florida to get on their surgical waiting list.

Surgery and Selecting a Surgeon

Okay, you have excess calcium disease. You want to be cured by having the calcium gland tumor(s) removed by surgery. You want to have this surgery very soon. What to do next?

Types of Surgery

For brevity, this book will present only three types of surgery—the two described in the mainstream medical websites (in the chapter "Monitoring or Surgery?") and Norman Center surgery. Let's start with the new material.

Norman Center Surgery

On the day of my surgery in Tampa, Dr. Norman wrote a letter to my (former) doctor and described my surgery as follows.[6] "Today we performed a Minimally Invasive Radioguided Calcium Gland Surgery . . . on [Peter] (an operation that we developed).[7] This is a simple out-patient procedure that includes the measurement of calcium hormone production from all four calcium glands (individually) in real-time." His letter continued: "Peter had a classic lower left calcium gland tumor (see actual size photo). The other three glands were anatomically normal and physiologically dormant." He concluded: "The entire procedure was uneventful and was completed in only 17 minutes. He went home about 1.5 hours later doing very well."

Mainstream Medical Surgery Options

The two types of surgery described on the mainstream medical websites were discussed earlier. A so-called "bilateral neck exploration" requires a 2" to 5" incision, perhaps 3 to 5 hours, and a possible hospital stay of one or two nights. While this type of surgery has the advantage of checking all four calcium glands (absolutely essential to be certain of a cure), the disadvantages are obvious (long scar, lengthy operation with increased risk and expense, etc.) A

6 The wording in the following letter has been changed to reflect the definitions used in this book so medical terms are replaced with layman's terms.

7 For purposes of this book, the operation performed as a matter of routine at the Norman Center will be referred to as "Norman Center surgery," not a "Minimally Invasive Radioguided Calcium Gland Surgery" or a "Minimally Invasive Radioguided Parathyroidectomy."

"minimally invasive" mainstream surgery is a much shorter outpatient procedure designed to remove a single calcium gland tumor (to be located by preoperative imaging).[8]

And the Winner Is . . .

Lengthy analysis is not necessary. The advantages of the Norman Center surgery, an outpatient sub-20 minute operation that checks all four calcium glands in real-time and removes all calcium gland tumors, are obvious. The only real disadvantages are the $1750 consultation fee and travel to Tampa, Florida for the operation.

Real World Experience

My operation at the Norman Center, described above, lasted 17 minutes, checked all four calcium glands, and left no scar. As described below, Carolyn and Walter had much different surgical experiences elsewhere. More information on my surgery appears later in this chapter.

8 Or there is the Mayo Clinic's "multiple incisions" for more than one calcium gland tumor.

Carolyn's Surgery

I sent Carolyn a list of questions about her diagnosis and surgery. She responded at length, for which I am grateful.

Carolyn's high blood calcium was discovered during a full physical. (Her symptoms, more fully described elsewhere, consisted primarily of very heavy fatigue and persistent urinary tract infections.) Her blood test results starred calcium as "high." Her calcium level was 11.1 and her lab report showed a normal range up to 10.2.

Carolyn went on the Internet the same day she received her blood test results and read that "your calcium level should never be high." The next day she contacted her doctor. Carolyn's PCP was also inclined to think she had excess calcium disease and Carolyn had a calcium hormone blood test that same day. When her PTH level was also high, the diagnosis of high calcium disease was made.

Next Carolyn was referred to an endocrinologist. (She did not see her PCP again.) The endocrinologist did not order more tests, confirmed the diagnosis, and immediately put her in touch with the surgeon in her HMO who did this type of surgery. Because the surgeon wanted to use an operating room with equipment to measure PTH levels during surgery and because another surgeon in the HMO wanted to assist, nothing happened for three months. As Carolyn was preparing for the wedding of her only daughter, these delays must have been stressful.

In her words, "preceding the surgery, I had extensive neck X-rays. The machine was large and took photos from many angles. It seemed long and very thorough.

Unfortunately, they didn't locate the tumor." Then her doctors had Carolyn take an MRI of the neck area. "The doctor did not readily see the tumor, but the technician pointed out what she thought it might be and the doctor agreed. They were not totally convinced but it gave the surgeons important information (they told me this after the surgery)." She was told that the surgery would take place even if the tumor could not located with imaging beforehand.

Carolyn's surgery finally occurred four weeks before her daughter's wedding. She had a fairly long incision horizontally across her neck. Four years after surgery, she is not unhappy with the scar—"a slim white line remains. Hard to see."

Both surgeons came to see her after surgery. They seemed proud of their "discovery and removal" of the tumor. "They said the second X-ray [MRI? sestamibi scan?] proved to be very helpful and told me how large it was in cm, but I don't recall. I asked if they kept it for me and they said no. They told me how quickly my [PTH] levels returned to normal."

Carolyn does not know if all four of her calcium glands were checked. She does not recall any discussion of checking all four glands. From her answers, it appears that the surgeons were satisfied that the high calcium disease was cured by the removal of one tumor because her PTH levels returned to normal during the operation. Again, the surgery was delayed and moved so it could be performed with equipment to measure the PTH level during the operation.

Carolyn's post-surgery recovery was joyful and will be described in a later chapter. Suffice to say that her daughter's wedding went off without a hitch. Carolyn is very satisfied with the medical care she received.

Walter's Surgery

Walter is a 60ish salesman of a high end product. He also responded to a list of questions from me, which I much appreciate. Walter went to the finest schools and is comfortable on both coasts. When calcium gland surgery was finally recommended, he was very careful. Like many of us, Walter uses his voice to earn a living. He was very concerned that if the surgery damaged his vocal cords, he would no longer be able to work.

By the time Walter had surgery, his calcium level exceeded 12.0. Interestingly, his PTH level was "about 60" or just above the high end of the normal range on lab test results. (Recall that 20% of excess calcium disease sufferers do not have an elevated PTH level.)

Walter endured three years of high calcium before surgery. He blames his internist for the long delay in diagnosis.[9] When he was finally referred to an endocrinologist, that specialist recommended monitoring and bisphosphonates (drugs used to treat osteoporosis [brittle bones]). By now, Walter knew enough about high

9 In addition to high calcium, Walter had elevated albumin. The reader of this book does not need to know what albumin is. (A visit to Wikipedia will not help.)

calcium disease to be shocked at this proposed course of treatment. He abandoned his local medical care, consulted an endocrinologist on the other coast, and eventually selected what he considered to be a highly qualified surgeon.

Walter's calcium gland surgery was performed in a teaching hospital by the head of surgery. His incision was small; he has no scar on his neck. Walter was given the option to remain conscious during surgery and chose to do so. (Both Carolyn and I were happy to be put under during surgery.)

My recollection of his oral account of the surgery is not perfect, but this is the gist of what Walter told me. Awake and conscious enough to communicate, Walter remembers the surgeon saying that he had found a tumor on the first calcium gland checked. Walter remembers the surgeon saying there was also a tumor on the second calcium gland checked. After a short delay, however, the surgeon returned and told Walter that there must be another tumor (or tumors) because his PTH level had not decreased to the normal range. At this point, Walter asked to be "put under" for the remainder of the surgery. And he was.

When Walter awoke, he learned from his surgeon that three of his four calcium glands had tumors and were removed. Fortunately his fourth calcium gland was normal. (Calcium glands are so important that nature provides them in quadruplicate—we only need one to function properly but we are given four to be certain that we have one that works.)

Walter had undergone sophisticated imaging tests before his operation but the results had not shown multiple calcium gland tumors. Walter's surgery lasted three to four hours. (In fact, all remaining surgeries on the day of Walter's surgery were delayed by several hours to await the completion of his operation.) He spent that night in the hospital and did not return home for another two days afterwards.

It is unclear exactly what label to place on Walter's surgery. It seems highly likely that his surgeon had not expected to inspect all four calcium glands during the operation. The fact that Walter was given the option to stay conscious during what turned into a three to four hour operation and the delays in the remainder of the day's surgical schedule indicate his surgeon expected to check and remove only one or perhaps two calcium glands, not all four.

Walter's post-surgery recovery is even more remarkable than Carolyn's and is discussed in the next chapter. Walter is unhappy with his medical care because of the delay in diagnosis but very happy with his surgeon. He believes his prudence in locating what he considered one of the finest surgeons in the U.S. was rewarded.

I am less sure. From their track record and the number of calcium gland surgeries they perform daily and weekly, I would be surprised if it took the surgeons at the Norman Center more than 30 minutes to perform Walter's operation. Calcium gland surgery is all they do and they encounter patients with tumors on three of the four calcium glands many times a month. NC blog, 6/8/13.

My Surgical Experience

Before Christmas vacation, 2013, I scheduled surgery at the Norman Parathyroid Center for Tuesday, January 28, 2014. I was to fly from Honolulu to Tampa leaving Sunday evening, January 26. I had a cold the week before departure and worried that I would not be able to fly, but departed on schedule. After flying all night, I arrived in Tampa early Monday afternoon and checked into the Westin Hotel about 2 pm. I ate dinner next door. I fell asleep about 4 am (11 pm in Hawaii) and awoke at 8:45 am on Tuesday morning.

I was fifteen minutes early for my 9:45 am appointment. The Medicare and insurance paperwork went smoothly. I met Dr. Politz, who gave me three sheets of paper to read and made it clear I must digest them before surgery. I found them sobering. They detailed what I would feel like after surgery and warned of the dangers of not enough calcium in the 10 days after the operation, hormonal changes likely, and the process of going from a life with too much calcium to a normal life. (For more detail, see next chapter.) One paper suggested taking it easy after surgery and said it was okay to go back to your room, nap for 3 or 4 hours, and then have soup in your room. "After all, you've had quite a day," it said.

The nurses were very professional and helpful. No problems inserting needles for an IV, etc. I got some help putting on a hospital gown. Kept valuables with me. After a time, I was taken off to nuclear medicine for a sestimibi scan. This involved lying flat on my back, completely still (could swallow as needed) after nuclear dye was injected into my body. It was okay to fall asleep during this, but I could not. During the third of four scans, I needed to scratch my nose, but the "crisis" passed. I never saw the results of these scans and did not ask about them.

Back in my pre-op location, I saw the couple who had checked in just before me. To my surprise, the wife was having the operation, not the husband. I don't know why I assumed it was him, not her. She looked very charged up to get it done (young woman, maybe 50, attractive, obviously looking forward to it).

My pre-operative visit with Dr. Norman was memorable. I liked the man a lot. He was very sincere. No trace of "been there, done that" 15,000 times. When he approached and introduced himself, I said I was dozing because of the time change from Hawaii and I admired the work he was doing. He said, "I'm a big fish in a small pond."

Picking up my file, he looked at me and said, "You have had this tumor for 8 to 10 years and it has ruined your life." Boom! Right out of the box. What took me by surprise was the 8 to 10 years part. I had assumed I got the tumor in early 2011, perhaps, and it had grown in 2012 and 2013. Nope. Had it 8 to 10 years. (I was so shocked by this that I did not focus on "and it has ruined your life" until that night, back in the hotel room). When the surgery was over and I saw a photo of my tumor (a photo is taken routinely), I was surprised at its size (not as large as expected given how high my calcium levels were) and the relatively low flow rate of calcium hormone (PTH flow was 650, which is ten times what it should be, but

PTH flow can go up to 2500). Dr. Politz dropped by after surgery. Still not convinced how long I had suffered from high calcium disease, I asked him how old he thought the tumor was. "Six years," he said. Later I repeated the question and Dr. Politz' answer to Dr. Norman. "Nope," he said, 8 to 10 years old because "it was very firm [hard]."

Back to the pre-op visit. I recall telling Dr. Norman two things before surgery. It took him a while to understand that I spent summers in the San Juan Islands in Washington state and winters in Hawaii. He approved (as do all men). Then I said in abbreviated fashion that I owned 10 acres of forest and spent my summers working outdoors with my dog and a chainsaw. I had done hard physical labor on my land for more than ten years. But by last summer (2013), I had not lifted a single piece of firewood. Dr. Norman was way ahead of me on this—I came to understand that his "and it has ruined your life" comment meant he knew what my story was going to be because it is not possible to have high calcium disease for 8 to 10 years without very serious impacts on daily life. After I said that last summer I didn't lift any firewood at all, he said "What I hate about this disease is that it removes the joy from life." By "ruined your life," he meant excess calcium disease removes all joy from life. This was not specific to me—it is common to all patients he sees who have had untreated high calcium disease for an extended time. Gracious!

The second thing I told Dr. Norman was that I had been going to my PCP for 15 years and my doctor "just missed it." I told him I later had met a woman on a cruise who had the operation and she told me about excess calcium disease. When I said I was the only person she had ever met who had high calcium disease and vice versa, **Dr. Norman said that 3 out of 4 women who have excess calcium disease do not know it.** He added that 1 in 80 women have high calcium disease. (The voiceover in the Norman Center video lists 1 in 850 people with a ratio of 3 women to every man; the graphics in the video have been updated to reflect these new numbers. See the transcript of the video in Chapter 1.)

As he was ready to leave, Dr. Norman said that I would be next, operation number 9 on the day. As I waited, I saw other patients in the pre-op area who were to follow me.

Soon a tall, very attractive female anesthesiologist came by, allowed me to go to the bathroom one last time, and then said she was going to get me ready for surgery. I mentioned a colonoscopy and she said those involve general anesthesia where they put you completely under. "I'm just going to make you loopy," she said. I think she was joking because I went under right then and remember nothing until a nurse woke me up 2.5 hours later. I am certain she woke me up, too, as I doubt I would have awakened on my own until I had caught up on about 12 hours of sleep.

After being awakened, I had three cups of coffee. It was 4 pm and I had been without food or liquid all day. I had the conversations with Politz and Norman described above, and I don't really recall anything else.

The Norman Center will not permit flights home on the day of surgery, so I went back to the Westin. As I lay in bed hoping to fall asleep (but not worrying about it), I realized my mind was different. The flow of excess calcium had been shut off. My mind was clearer, sharper, than I could remember for a very long time. (Continued in the next chapter.)

How to Pick a Surgeon

What do we make of these three different surgical experiences? All three patients are happy, even thrilled, with the outcome of surgery. Carolyn views her surgery on the eve of her daughter's wedding as one of the best things to happen to her in her life. Walter was astonished by the post-surgery enhancement of his senses. He could see better, hear better, taste better. While my results were more subdued, I am pleased with the long-term results of my surgery.

Each operation was successful. Yet each operation was different.

Carolyn had what appears to be a "bilateral neck exploration" with a long scar but she is not certain that all four calcium glands were checked. Even though it may not have been the original intent, Walter is certain that all four of his glands were checked because three of them were removed! And he has no scar. But Walter's operation lasted three to four hours and required an overnight stay in the hospital. My surgery was cookie-cutter Norman Center outpatient surgery lasting 17 minutes.

There is a lesson here. If calcium gland surgery is successful, whether it is performed by a very experienced surgeon who does many such operations daily or weekly (Norman Center) or by a highly skilled surgeon who does not do as many (Walter's doctor at a teaching hospital) or by the local HMO surgeon who has done "many" but not a large number of such surgeries (and leaves a scar), patients who are cured are happy. Better an imperfect surgery (long operation, scar) than none at all.

There is useful information available on-line to help a person with high calcium disease choose a surgeon. Most of the following advice comes from the Norman Center website. As we review it, there will be instances where the surgeries performed on Carolyn and Walter will appear not to be what we might call "best practices." But don't tell that to Carolyn or Walter; they will not care.

Dr. Norman's Advice on Selecting a Surgeon

While reading the advice from Dr. Norman that follows, keep in mind that his foremost concern is that any calcium gland surgery **should check all four calcium glands**. His harshest criticisms are aimed at surgical practices that he views as excuses for failure to check all four glands. (Surgeons do not check all four calcium glands because it typically takes them 2 to 5 hours to do so.) NC blog, 11/24/13.

For a time, the Norman Center surgeons checked only two of the four glands during a calcium gland operation. We will call this "unilateral" surgery, checking only the two glands on one side of the neck. Later the Norman Center surgeons also performed "bilateral" surgery, checking all four glands. When the cure rates were compared, bilateral surgery was the clear winner. In an October, 2011 presentation to the American College of Surgeons, Drs. Norman, Politz, and Lopez from the Norman Center recommended "bilateral" surgery (checking all four glands). "Allowing rapid analysis of all 4 glands through the same 1-inch incision has caused us to all but abandon unilateral [surgery]." Journal of the American College of Surgeons, March, 2012, Volume 214, Issue 3, Pages 260-269.

Up to 30% of people with high calcium disease have more than one calcium gland tumor. 2% of patients have 3 tumors. 3% of patients have 4 tumors. NC blog, 6/8/13.[10] A cure is complete and permanent only when surgery removes all calcium gland tumors. Unless all calcium gland tumors are removed, high calcium disease is not cured.

Nearly one in five calcium gland surgeries (eighteen percent) performed at the Norman Center is a second operation. NC blog, 9/20/13. That is, nearly one in five patients has already had a calcium gland operation (elsewhere) and it failed. Either the surgeon was not able to locate the single calcium gland tumor or the surgeon found one tumor, removed it, and then ended the operation without checking the other three glands. Ten percent of all calcium gland operations at the Norman Center are to remove a second tumor that was missed in the first operation. This appears to amount to half of the "second operations" performed.

---

10 A discussion of surgical techniques when four calcium tumors are present is beyond the scope of this book.

In the blog entry dated 9/20/13, Dr. Norman lists six reasons why excess calcium disease can be "very tricky."

1. There are 4 calcium glands and a person with high calcium disease can have 1, 2, 3, or all 4 bad glands.
2. At least 30% of people with excess calcium disease will have more than one bad calcium gland.
3. There is no test that can tell a surgeon before the operation whether the patient has only one or more than one calcium gland tumor.
4. There is no test that can tell a surgeon during the operation whether the patient has only one or more than one calcium gland tumor.
5. Normal calcium glands are the size of a grain of rice.
6. Although normally found near the thyroid, calcium glands can be found anywhere from high under the jaw to low down in the chest next to the heart.

If you analyze these six issues, each one either counters "expert advice" that it is not necessary to check all four glands during the operation or explains why your surgeon never found the calcium gland tumor.

Dr. Norman also lists 8 red flags that a surgeon is not (or was not) experienced enough to perform calcium gland surgery (same blog).

1. Removing [single] calcium gland tumor that shows on preoperative scan and then ending operation (need to check all 4).
2. Performing a different calcium gland operation if preoperative imaging is positive [shows tumor] vs. negative [does not show a tumor].

(The Norman Center uses scans only to locate ectopic calcium glands.)

3. Operating on only one side of neck (unilateral surgery) so not checking 2 glands on other side (bilateral surgery).
4. Making an incision off to side of neck instead of middle (need to check all 4 glands).
5. Operating only when scan is positive [shows tumor] (scan is not reliable prediction tool).
6. Using words like "focused, targeted, specific" because implies all 4 glands won't be checked.
7. Using larger, bigger incision in order to check all 4 glands [leaving a scar].
8. Failing to examine all 4 glands.

A Ninth Red Flag: Looking for 50% drop in PTH value during operation

This last blog entry should have added a ninth red flag, to wit:

9. Measuring PTH level during operation and pretending patient is cured if PTH level drops in value by 50%, rather than checking all 4 glands. Dr. Norman is so opposed to this practice, which he believes to be an excuse to not check all four glands, that he labels it as **"the biggest crock of crap ever propagated by surgeons on their unsuspecting patients."** [emphasis added] (same blog)

The Norman Center does about 2600 calcium gland surgeries per year. "We have the best technology and enough money to buy any new technology that we need or want. If measuring PTH in the operating room worked and had value, then we would do it. We do not." NC blog, 6/8/13. Dr. Norman continues: "We cannot have people travelling hundreds or thousands of miles and not be cured. The ONLY way to assure very high cure rates (over 90% theoretically and 99% in our case) is to see all four calcium glands in all patients. This is what we do." [emphasis in original] (same blog)

The NC blog entry continues: "If these surgeons tell you that they measure the PTH in the operating room and that will give a cure rate of 99% or better without looking at all four calcium glands, then they are not being honest with you. That simply is not possible. **Be smart and remember there is no 'doctor police.' Doctors can say and do anything they want . . . and they do.**" [emphasis added] (same blog)

The NC blog entry of 11/13/13 finishes the point. "Folks, we do NOT use intra-operative PTH monitoring because **it does not work** . . . ." [emphasis in original] "Virtually every [second operation] patient we operate on (2-3 per day) had a surgeon use PTH monitoring in the operating room INSTEAD of looking at all 4 calcium glands. If measuring PTH in the operating room worked, we would do it!" [emphasis in original] (same blog)

Never Allow Your Surgeon to use a Scope

Perhaps the worst thing that can happen during calcium gland surgery is for the tumor to be punctured or severed during removal so that it spills or spreads calcium hormone into the surrounding parts of the body. "A broken calcium gland tumor can be a devastating complication of surgery. Calcium gland tumor cells will grow almost anywhere, so they must not be broken during surgery. Calcium gland tumor implants are very hard to cure." NC blog, 8/14/13. One of the most important rules of excess calcium disease surgery is **"do not break the calcium gland tumor; it must be removed from the patient's neck completely intact."** [emphasis in original] (same blog).

The Norman Center very strongly advises against attempts to remove calcium gland tumors located in the chest through a scope. "We have seen 6 patients who will never be cured of excess calcium disease because their surgeon tried to remove [an ectopic calcium gland located in the chest] with a scope. They broke the tumor and pieces of it grew all over their chest cavity and lungs. Some of the worst cases we have ever seen are because of broken chest tumors—broken by surgeons using scopes in the chest." NC blog, 8/5/13.

In the view of the Norman Center surgeons, almost all calcium gland tumors in the chest (ectopic tumors) can be removed through a small neck incision . . . provided your surgeon knows how to do it. **Less than 5% of chest calcium gland tumors require a "chest" operation to remove it . . . .**" [emphasis in original] (same blog). For ectopic tumors deep in the chest, the Norman Center schedules a "chest Wednesday" with a heart surgeon about once every three months. No scopes are used in the surgery.

Action Items for Readers

1. Get surgery as fast as you can but carefully question your surgeon before selecting him or her.
2. Be most concerned that your surgeon will check each of the four calcium glands during the operation. Do not accept any surgical technique that attempts to substitute for checking all four glands.
3. Be certain your operation proceeds rapidly regardless of the results of preoperative imaging or scans, if any.
4. If you have ectopic glands (shown on preoperative images), strongly consider starting at the Norman Center because you may end up in Tampa for a second operation anyway.
5. In general, do not be afraid to self-refer to the surgeon of your choice, including the Norman Center in Tampa, if you can afford it. Remember that Medicare and/or private health insurance will cover the costs of surgery wherever it takes place.

Post-surgery Experience

Successful calcium gland surgery, defined as removal of all calcium gland tumors, cures the disease. Completely. One hundred percent. The life of a patient who undergoes successful surgery is improved. Always. Before we turn to how individual lives have been improved, let us review some general health statistics.

Improvement in Overall Health

Remember the transcript of the voiceover of the Norman Center video on high calcium disease? Recall this statement: "It is estimated that untreated excess calcium disease can decrease a patient's life expectancy by 5 or 6 years even when the calcium is only slightly elevated." This health risk goes away with successful surgery.

More specific statistics are available. The Norman Center blog of 6/23/13 states that when the calcium gland tumor is removed and the high calcium disease is cured, the risk for breast cancer decreases within a year or two, the risk for kidney stones and kidney failure decreases dramatically within hours, the blood flow through the coronary arteries increases within weeks, cardiac muscle contraction increases within weeks, the risk of bone fractures decreases within months, and on and on.

The same blog lists citations to numerous scholarly medical articles that document the positive consequences of successful calcium gland surgery. The 41 medical journal articles list in an understated way the benefits of surgery, including: (2) A strong correlation exists between breast cancer and excess calcium disease, (24) surgery for high calcium disease "seems to reduce both systolic and diastolic blood pressure," (33) "Depression, anxiety, and decreased Quality of Life appear related to the [disease]." Successful surgery "seems to reduce psychopathologic symptoms and improve Quality of Life in this setting."

According to Item 28 on the list, after surgery prescription drugs taken by patients "should be routinely reviewed and adjusted . . . anticipating elimination of some." This certainly applied to me. In two post-surgery visits to my new doctor, my blood pressure had decreased so dramatically that I proposed cutting my blood pressure medications in half, to which my new doctor immediately agreed.

Case Studies on the Norman Center Blog

Individual case studies provide examples of dramatic improvements in health following successful surgery.

Excess calcium disease in pregnant women can cause miscarriages. The Norman Center blog entry of 5/17/13 describes a 30-year-old female with high blood calcium of 11.7 mg/dl. (identical to mine). 20 weeks pregnant and with a history of miscarriages, she was referred by her obstetrician in Los Angeles. The blog reviews the relationship between miscarriages and high calcium disease and concludes, "high calcium is a real and direct threat to the baby." The woman had a routine operation (no sestamibi scan because of the pregnancy) and was discharged in 2.5 hours total. After the operation, the baby was carried to full term. As the couple had suffered several miscarriages, the birth of an 8 lb. 7 oz. girl brought great joy.

Although no other case study described in the Norman Center blog contains this much joy, all of them end on a positive note. The patients described in the blog entries typically experience a significant reduction in their most troublesome symptoms.

While my post-surgery experience has been satisfactory, it has not reached the level of rosiness and bliss presented in the case studies of the blog patients. But I may be the exception that proves the rule. The post-surgery histories of Carolyn and Walter make the recoveries of the Norman Center blog patients appear understated in comparison.

Carolyn's Wedding

At dinner on the cruise ship, I was struck by Carolyn's ecstatic description of how much better she felt immediately after surgery. Immediately meant right away—no delay at all! Perhaps this happened because her only daughter's wedding was just four weeks away, but from the day of surgery onward, she had her old energy and enthusiasm back. Her husband, Dave, agreed wholeheartedly with this description.

When she suffered from high calcium disease, Carolyn had difficulty going on even short walks with her husband. On one outing with Dave, she burst into tears when she realized how much further she had to walk to return to the starting point. On the ship, she had no difficulty with their daily deck walking (and they got in over 10,000 steps a day!). She looks back on her pre-surgery self with sympathy and regret. Carolyn is pleased that she was able to tell me about excess calcium disease and looks forward to a much wider understanding of the disease.

Walter's Senses

Walter's post-operative experience was even more profound than Carolyn's. Walter had been under heavy calcium assault for more than three years. Without realizing it, he had gradually lost the full range of his senses—vision, hearing, smell, and taste. By the time he returned home from surgery, he understood just how much he had been missing.

When Walter first awoke from surgery, he was surprised to be able to hear two nurses talking at a substantial distance from him. They were not talking loudly—this was a recovery room in a hospital after all. But he could hear them clearly. This surprised him enormously.

Walter flies often. He has a favorite airline and a favorite flight time and he usually ends up near the same gates at the airport. When he deplaned from his return flight after surgery, Walter could smell hamburgers cooking at a McDonald's near his gate. It was a penetrating smell, but he could not remember ever smelling it before. He wondered why not.

When he arrived at his house, Walter decided to have a bottle of wine to celebrate. Walter considers himself an oenophile, a connoisseur of fine wines, yet when he opened one of his favorite bottles, it tasted much different from what he remembered. It was still good, but not what he was used to. This was true of the next bottle he opened and the next. In this fashion, Walter discovered that his sense of taste had returned. The desire for VERY spicy foods, "in some cases so hot that nobody else could eat them," disappeared. His taste buds worked normally again.

His vision improved, too. Walter lives in a sunny place. Before surgery, he usually drove his car without sunglasses, something almost unheard of in his area. If he drove into an indoor parking garage with sunglasses on, it would be too dark to see. After surgery, this changed. He could no longer drive without sunglasses and he could see just fine inside indoor parking garages even wearing sunglasses.

In Walter's words, "I had a gradual reduction in sensory perception across all senses but was not aware of it because it had declined so gradually. I only became aware of it after surgery." He was aware of odd behavior in himself (sunglasses, spicy foods), "but had not connected the dots."

After surgery, everything became clear. Walter estimates that his senses were impaired or reduced by about 30%. Walter will tell you that he can see, hear, taste, and smell 30 to 40 percent better than before surgery. To him, this borders on miraculous.

One of the Norman Center's blog patients had an experience similar to Walter's. Dr. Goyal, the family care doctor who had calcium gland surgery himself in Tampa after one of his patients self-referred to the Norman Center, submitted a long list of his improvements post-surgery. As summarized from the NC blog dated 10/12/13, at "one month post surgery:"

1. Had large tumor, despite negative scans.
2. Feel younger.
3. More alert, more focused, very energetic, very motivated to work.
4. Don't feel depressed like I used to. Not anxious. Not tired or lazy.
5. Sleep meds reduced by 80%.
6. Hair returning to scalp, thicker.
7. Sunken cheeks have filled out. Wife says I look younger and healthier.
8. Open my eyes wider (physically). Right eye, am able to focus more.
9. Ears: Can now hear far away music volumes [better] than before. Lowered TV volume by at least 60%.
10. Nose: I can smell so much better now. Now I have to clean all the bad smells in the house daily.

11. Speech. Has become so much stronger. I had been losing speech for last 3 years.
12. Lungs: Breathing is deeper again. Finally I can meditate better, which I had been struggling with for last 4 years.
13. Blood pressure. Have decreased my medication 20% in one month.
14. Bones. Never had bone pain.
15. Joints. Shoulder and hip joints are loosened up and flexing again. Happy about this.
16. Exercise. I'm in the gym regularly and use 20 to 40 lbs. extra on other machines. My stamina has increased by 60%.
17. Napping and tiredness. I used to lie down in bed for short nap several times a day but not any more.

Dr. Goyal chronicled these improvements only one month post-surgery! Is it any wonder that people who hear a description of high calcium disease say (or think) "I hope I have this disease?"

Range of Post-Operative Responses

When I had my surgery at the Norman Center, I knew only about Carolyn's post-surgery experience. It is a good thing that I did not meet Walter until later because my expectations were already too high.

On the morning of my surgery I checked into the Norman Center on the sixth floor of Tampa General Hospital.

I was immediately given a two-page handout titled "What to Expect Today and in the Coming Weeks." The handout contained an instructive and restrained description of what to expect post surgery. (This book will ignore the portion devoted to day of surgery expectations and activities.)

Longer term, the Norman Center handout stated: "Keep in mind the rabbit and the tortoise. People recover at different rates. The rabbit peels out right out of the gate (the patient who feels fantastic the very next morning and can't wait to tell the world how great they are doing!). They run way ahead of the pack, and when they get near the finish line, they are the loudest and the happiest . . . good for them." This is Carolyn's experience. Right?

The handout continues: "Most patients ('the pack') will notice the difference somewhere around two weeks after having a tumor removed. They are not way up front with the rabbit, but they're surely not trailing way behind the pack where the tortoise is. There is nothing wrong with you if you are in the pack." This is Walter's experience, more or less. After his calcium gland surgery, Walter spent a night in the hospital and then another two days resting before he flew home. It took him several days to recognize the depth of his sensory improvements. Still, his recovery seems relatively fast.

And the tortoise? As described in the Norman Center handout, "The tortoise is going to get there, too. He's just going to take his sweet time (maybe 6-8 weeks). So don't panic if you don't wake up a completely new person the morning after the tumor is removed. Most people don't." This was my experience, except possibly I was a "super tortoise."

My Post-Op Experience

I had to fly a very long distance from Hawaii to Tampa. To do so, I cashed in 60,000 airline miles for a free round trip ticket. This got me coach seats on the two legs going to Tampa (through Houston) and on those two legs I paid extra for "economy plus" (more legroom, etc.) My cashed miles enabled me to fly business class on the longest leg back to Hawaii (Houston to Honolulu) and I upgraded to first class from Tampa to Houston. I figured, rightly, that I would need to take care of myself post-surgery.

After flying all night to get to Tampa, I arrived the afternoon before my surgery and tried to acclimate to the five-hour time change from Hawaii. I was able to get about four hours of sleep.

My surgical experience at the Norman Center inside the Tampa General Hospital was entirely satisfactory. I left my hotel about 9:30 am and returned in late afternoon after surgery. Unable to nap, I ordered room service for dinner and was again unable to sleep. The next morning I checked out at 4:30 am for an early departure back to Hawaii. My flights were on time and comfortable, but I did not sleep. On arrival in Honolulu, I was pretty much dead meat.

Contrary to Carolyn's experience of hitting the ground running the day after surgery, overall I felt worse after surgery because of lack of sleep, time changes, and long flights. It took several days to make up the missed sleep. Whatever the reason, I never felt even an iota of the "renewed energy" that Carolyn relished or the increased sensory pleasures that Walter welcomed back into his life.

The "tortoise or hare" handout gave me reassurance that things would get better. The handout continues: "Certain symptoms get better at different times. Memory loss, mental sharpness, energy levels, concentration abilities, mood stability—these things typically start to get better between 8 and 14 days on average. Some people don't feel better for a month or two." It continues: "Think about it. Your nervous system has to get used to a normal calcium level again. Your brain has not seen normal calcium levels for years. Remember, this disease occurred over a period of years; some things will take months to get better."

While it took me many months to improve significantly, I did have one Carolyn or Walter-like experience. In the pre-operative visit Dr. Norman said to me "You have had this disease for 8 to 10 years and it has ruined your life." My one "eureka" experience involved mental puzzle solving based on this statement. When I got back to my hotel room (and was unable to sleep), my mind, on its own, decided to analyze the new information that I had suffered from excess calcium disease for 8 to 10 years. Pretty much beyond my control, my mind reviewed my history over the last 8 to 10 years to evaluate my behavior in light of this new information. It was an intense and startling mental experience. As it was happening, I was aware that regardless of the validity of any conclusions reached, I had not had a mental experience of such complexity and depth in many, many years. It was like Walter hearing the nurses from far away. Long time, no experience. Welcome back.

Building upon that mental exercise, I decided to write to my ex-wife and two daughters to attempt to explain some of what I had learned about excess calcium disease and how long I had endured it. At the six-week point post-surgery, I sent such a letter off. At that time, I proclaimed myself to be a tortoise. As more time has passed, I consider myself to be a super-tortoise, taking three or four months or longer to "return to normal."

After his surgery, Walter faulted himself for failing to "connect the dots" and to realize something significant had been wrong with him. It was not until I wrote this book that I went through a similar "why didn't I connect the dots" analysis.

I had three red flag incidents that should have triggered a realization that something was really wrong. The first occurred in the fall of 2011, more than two years before surgery, when I suffered a massive muscle pull in the back of my left leg. This happened while I was lying in bed doing a morning stretch (a "glad to be alive" full body stretch before getting up). Because it was on the back of my leg (and I was living alone), I did not see the half-watermelon sized bruise that resulted. It was brought to my attention only when I went to my doctor's office for another reason. I was immediately sent for x-rays and imaging, but my doctor never could figure out why a simple morning stretch would cause such an injury.

Eight months after this muscle pull, in June of 2012, I moved into my newly constructed house in the San Juan Islands. I rented a Penske truck, loaded my household belongings, and, with help from a lovely woman, spent the day unloading things into my new 1000 sq. ft. house. That evening, I took the truck off the island on a barge, turned it back in without refueling it (too tired to remember), and drove a car to SeaTac airport where I was to pick up my daughter and her boyfriend early the next morning. When I finally got to bed at a Motel 6 that night, my quads in both legs knotted up so completely that I was unable to move. I remember thinking, "If I could reach my cell phone, I would call 911 and go to the hospital." I could not move at all, so I could not reach my cell phone. When these massive muscle spasms finally eased, I did not call 911. Instead I drank lots of water and tried to remain completely still for the rest of the night. These were extraordinarily painful muscle spasms, but it did not occur to me that anything was out of the ordinary.

During the summer of 2013 (described to my physician as "bad" at my physical that fall), I failed to notice a paper wasp's nest. My island house is a one-story affair with a slightly raised ceiling (11' at the peak). One can enter through a sliding glass door off the kitchen to a 5' wide deck. All summer long I entered and exited through the sliding glass door many times a day. By now I napped each afternoon and generally dragged around. Somehow I never looked up to see a paper wasp's nest being built above the deck. Shaped like a football standing upright in a kicking tee, it was about twice the size of a football and home to hundreds of wasps. One afternoon I had the sensation a bee flying near my hair. When I looked up, I was shocked to see a paper wasp's nest with countless wasps flying in or out of the bottom of the nest.

When I finally noticed them, the wasps ignored me. Although the main purpose of "soldier" wasps is to attack any enemy of the nest, I had been around so long that I was "natural" and part of the landscape. They were used to me, even if I had failed to notice hundreds of them right outside my kitchen door (and clearly visible through my kitchen window). One can use words to describe chronic fatigue (feeling tired all the time) but to me, the paper wasp's nest exemplifies excess calcium disease.[11]

So, who should feel worse about failing to connect the dots? Walter? Or me?

The Recovery Path

Mental

The two main aspects of returning to normal are physical and mental. As to mental, I believe that for life to be satisfying and enjoyable, one has to accomplish things. Without my awareness, high calcium disease established what for me were insurmountable barriers to accomplishments.

I have been a self-starter all my life. I would often say to myself and others, "by such and such a time I am going to accomplish x, y, and z." And in my earlier life, I usually did. With excess calcium disease, at the end of

11 It was a lengthy adventure involving only a broom, but I got rid of the wasp's nest without a single sting!

such and such a time, not only had I not accomplished x or y or z, I had rarely even started one of them. When this failure happens repeatedly and one has no idea why, it is profoundly discouraging. Low mood? You bet. Depression? Nope, not me. Irritability? Yes. Fat and out of shape? Yes.

When calcium gland tumors are removed and calcium in the blood returns to normal, previously unknown impediments are removed. But accomplishments do not follow quickly or automatically. They take time and are built step by step. Even with perfect health, the bigger the goal, the bigger the task, the longer it takes to accomplish what one sets out to do.

As I reached the one-year anniversary of my surgery, I noticed accomplishments building up. In the decade of the 2000s, I spent almost six years writing a book about a plane crash and rescue on Mt. McKinley and a trial that followed. Unable to find a literary agent in 2008, I put the book aside. (This timing coincides with the onset of high calcium disease.) After my surgery, I picked the book up, revised it a final time, and self-published it under the title "*Denali Justice*" in the fall of 2014, nine months after surgery. I am pleased with the effort and if it ever becomes visible in the publishing world or on the Internet, I think sales will be good. In any event, I am proud of the accomplishment.

With one book published, I decided to write this book partly as a public service. If you are reading this, then I succeeded in publishing it. Another accomplishment.

In the months following surgery, I decided to become a bridge director (a person who runs card games). I found this rewarding. 8 months after surgery, I served as the bridge director on a Holland America cruise from Vancouver, BC to Sydney, Australia. During the cruise, I taught 15 well-attended bridge lessons to intermediate players and ran 15 large bridge games. I would not have been capable of this before the surgery.

Physical

The Norman Center handouts also focus on physical recovery. Calcium intake and regulation immediately post-surgery is an extremely important but temporary issue that is not within the scope of this book. (Pay strict attention to your post-surgery instructions!) What is within the scope of this book is the path towards rebuilding the physical well being of a person who has endured long-term excess calcium disease.

The Norman Center advises patients to take calcium supplements (two 630 mg caps per day with Vitamin D) for up to two years. A friend who is a general practice physician has told me he expects it to take 3 or 4 years for my bone and muscle strength to return fully. While I have been offered the name of an endocrinologist to measure my bone strength, I declined the referral. I understand the limitations regarding physical recovery and I am learning to be patient.

As quoted in the beginning of this book, in mid-October, 2013, I was in the worst physical shape of my life. Although, like Walter, I did not connect the dots, it is now clear that high calcium disease was to blame. As I wrote this book, I realized it had been several years since I indulged in a full-body, early morning, "glad to be alive" stretch like the one that resulted in the severe muscle pull in the fall of 2011. Basically I don't get enough physical exercise to induce a satisfying stretch. When my muscles and bones have rebuilt themselves, however, I look forward to a return of this morning ritual.

In the last two years before surgery, I performed very little physical work. My body was not capable of the usual work on the island where I live most of the year. For example, I heat my main house and guesthouse with wood stoves. This requires cutting up blown over trees, splitting the rounds, and carrying and stacking the split wood. This work stopped completely. As I told Dr. Norman on the day of my surgery, in the summer of 2013, I could not remember even picking up a piece of wood.

With surgery in January 2014 behind me, I resolved to improve my physical condition. I have been out of shape before (though never this bad) and have some experience with getting back into shape. My number one goal was to avoid what would have been my third bout of plantar fasciitis, a painful foot injury usually caused by going too quickly from not enough running to too much running. I resolved to increase the number of steps I walked gradually. (Aren't pedometers wonderful?)

I still went too fast. After easily building up my daily step count to 10,000, I went with friends to attend a music concert at a Buddhist temple on the windward side of Oahu. I strayed from the musical presentation and tried to walk around the temple building. While doing this, I got one foot caught in quicksand-like mud. As I extracted my foot, apparently I pulled or tore my quad muscle. Soon enough, I could barely walk. This lasted for months.

I also suffered from GERD-like symptoms. Some of the literature suggests that calcium gland surgery will resolve GERD symptoms after only one month, but I did not learn this until later. Immediately after surgery, I was advised by a friend that coffee can induce GERD so I gave up coffee and the GERD went away. To help with weight loss, I also stopped drinking alcohol. Three months later, when I resumed drinking coffee (and alcohol), my symptoms of GERD did not return.

It is not hard to listen to your body when you try and I am getting better at it. As a result, the summer of 2014 also passed with little or no wood being carried. It has now been over one year since my surgery and I feel better month-to-month. I expect to begin some real work in the summer of 2015. If this is too soon, I will back off and let my muscles and bones heal further. Just as mental accomplishments take time (writing a book), regaining physical strength when recovering from high calcium disease takes time. As long as the trend is in the right direction, I am happy.

Action Items for Readers

1. Manage your post surgery expectations. You might be a rabbit (yea!) but be prepared to be a tortoise.
2. Give yourself several weeks or months before you expect to feel significantly better.
3. Ease into physical conditioning. Your body has suffered damage that cannot be repaired as quickly as your mind.
4. Remember, you are cured. The disease does not return. Life gets better every day.

About the Author

Despite annual blood tests and medical exams, Peter A. Galbraith unknowingly suffered from excess calcium disease for over eight years before surgery in 2014. He is the author of *Denali Justice*.

Made in the USA
Charleston, SC
08 August 2016